S. Hrg. 105–45, Part I

PERSIAN GULF WAR ILLNESSES, PART I

HEARING

BEFORE THE

COMMITTEE ON VETERANS' AFFAIRS
UNITED STATES SENATE

ONE HUNDRED FIFTH CONGRESS

FIRST SESSION

JANUARY 9, 1997

Printed for the use of the Committee on Veterans' Affairs

U.S. GOVERNMENT PRINTING OFFICE

41-207 CC WASHINGTON : 1997

For sale by the U.S. Government Printing Office
Superintendent of Documents, Congressional Sales Office, Washington, DC 20402
ISBN 0-16-055298-2

COMMITTEE ON VETERANS' AFFAIRS

ARLEN SPECTER, Pennsylvania, *Chairman*

STROM THURMOND, South Carolina
FRANK H. MURKOWSKI, Alaska
JAMES M. JEFFORDS, Vermont
BEN NIGHTHORSE CAMPBELL, Colorado
LARRY E. CRAIG, Idaho
Y. TIM HUTCHINSON, Arkansas

JOHN D. ROCKEFELLER IV, West Virginia
BOB GRAHAM, Florida
DANIEL K. AKAKA, Hawaii
PAUL WELLSTONE, Minnesota
PATTY MURRAY, Washington

CHARLES BATTAGLIA, *Staff Director*
JIM GOTTLIEB, *Minority Chief Counsel/Staff Director*

CONTENTS

JANUARY 9, 1997

APPENDIX

PERSIAN GULF WAR VETERANS' ILLNESSES, PART I

THURSDAY, JANUARY 9, 1997

U.S. SENATE
COMMITTEE ON VETERANS' AFFAIRS
Washington, D.C.

The Committee met, pursuant to notice, at 9:38 a.m. in room 216, Hart Senate Office Building, Hon. Arlen Specter (Chairman of the Committee) presiding.

Present: Senators Specter, Jeffords, Hutchinson, Rockefeller, Wellstone, and Murray.

Chairman SPECTER. We're waiting for Senator Rockefeller. We know the snow conditions, so we'll just wait a moment or two until he arrives.

The hearing of the Veterans' Committee will now proceed.

OPENING STATEMENT OF CHAIRMAN SPECTER

This is the first Committee hearing of the Veterans' Committee in the 105th Congress. We have just been organized and, under the new Rules of the Senate, there is an election for Chairman, so I thank my colleagues for the election. Senator Rockefeller, our distinguished ranking member, and I have already consulted extensively on issues which the Committee will be looking into. We welcome Senator Hutchinson as a new member to our Committee.

Today we proceed with the issue of the Gulf War Syndrome. This is the first of a series of hearings which this Committee will have both here in Washington and in the field. The two major issues which we will be looking at, at least initially, relate to what happened to the Gulf War veterans, are they being adequately treated and compensated for their exposure to a variety of problems in the Gulf War; and the second issue, what action was taken by the Department of Defense, the other branches of Government to find out what happened, whether the veterans were exposed to chemical warfare, just exactly what occurred back at Khamisiyah in March 1991 when an Iraqi chemical compound was detonated, and why it was not made public until 1996.

As a personal note and some of my own background on approaching the issues of the veterans, the treatment accorded by the Federal Government, this has been a matter of long standing interest to me since I was a child. Just for a moment or two on a personal basis my own perspective. The first veteran I knew was Harry Specter, my father, who was a veteran in World War I. He was an immigrant from Russia, literally walked across Europe with barely a ruble in his pocket, came to America, did not know that he had a round trip ticket to France to the Argonne Forest where he served in World War I. He was inducted on May 6 of 1918 at Fairbury, Nebraska. He had left the East Coast and gone to the Midwest. He sailed for France on June 4 of 1918, 29 days after he was inducted. I've always wondered about the adequacy of his training; really cannon fodder right onto the battlefields in the Argonne Forest, where he was wounded in action.

My recollection is of his concerns and anger when the Federal Government reneged on the commitment to pay World War I veterans a bonus. They had the famous march. We lived in Wichita, Kansas. He could hardly join that march either geographically or physically, really. But I remember his chagrin at the failure of the Government to honor the payments of the bonus. In the Depression days, all that kept the wolf from the door in the Specter household was a small disability check. He was not given his bonus. And in a sense, and I've said this before but it's worth repeating, I think I've been on my way to Washington ever since to get my father's bonus check. So, when I see and hear what is happening on this Gulf War Syndrome, it is a matter of enormous concern.

We have a report of a distinguished presidential commission, and we're glad to have Dr. Joyce Lashof with us here today. Dr. Lashof spoke in a meeting with the President two days ago, Senator Rockefeller and I were present, and characterized the efforts by the Department of Defense as superficial, lacked credibility, failed to seriously investigate, and commented about the intransigence of the Department of Defense. Findings of the commission are voluminous, but just on two of them: "The evidence of chemical warfare agent release at Khamisiyah is overwhelming and low level exposure to troops within a fifty kilometer radius should be presumed." And, "DOD has conducted a superficial investigation of possible chemical warfare agent exposure that is unlikely to provide credible answers to veterans' and the public's questions."

The purpose of this oversight hearing, and others, will be to provide that kind of a response. General H. Norman Schwarzkopf characterized the Pentagon's handling of the issue in the first years after the war as "almost scandalous." There is a great deal more that could be said by way of introduction, but we will be developing precisely what happened. I have conferred with Secretary Brown who has pledged his full cooperation, met this morning with acting Director of the CIA George Tenet who is here to testify. The presidential commission compliments the CIA for the work which it has done. It's nice to have a public compliment occasionally. We will be working very hard on this matter.

I would like to yield now to my distinguished ranking member who has been in this field for a long while. In my capacity as Chairman of the Intelligence Committee, I initiated a joint hearing with the Veterans' Affairs Committee back on September 25 of last year. Just coincidentally, on the morning of our hearing the Deputy Secretary of Defense sent a letter to the Chairman of the Armed Services Committee for the first time saying that the Department of Defense would do a little something about this issue. I'm sure it was just coincidental that the letter came as we were conducting the hearing. I got it while Senator Rockefeller and I and others were here. But Senator Rockefeller wrote a very extensive letter following that hearing to the President and the Secretary of Defense. I yield now to Senator Rockefeller.

[The opening statement of Chairman Specter appears on page 50.]

OPENING STATEMENT OF SENATOR ROCKEFELLER

Senator ROCKEFELLER. Thank you, Chairman Specter. I apologize to the witnesses that there is always this matter of Senators making statements, but that's because it gives us a chance to say what we want to, not in question form, but declaratively, and set the tone.

First, I want to congratulate you, Chairman Specter. I can't tell you how much I look forward to working with you as Chairman. In the last couple of years, this Committee has been relatively dormant. I'm very confident that under you it will not be. You and I have very similar views on this subject, and I'm sure many others. So, your return to the Chairmanship is very welcome by this Democrat. I wish I were in your position, but I'm not. [Laughter.] That being the case, I'm very happy that you are. I also want to say that I look forward, as does Jim Gottlieb, my chief of staff, to working with your Chief of Staff, Charlie Battaglia. There's an excellent working relationship already.

I want to thank you, obviously, for calling today's hearing so early in the session. We both have a commitment to this. Most of us have come to acknowledge that a large number of previously very healthy men and women returned home from the Persian Gulf with a myriad of health complaints and illnesses. They started out—and I've seen scores of them—they started out healthy, and they came back sick. That's clear. In some cases, they have become greatly disabled, dysfunctional. That is clear. Nobody disputes that. In addition to the pain and the losses that our veterans have experienced in coping with the health problems that they're struggling to understand, they have also had to endure the humiliation of being told that their problems are not real. They continue to cope with the fear that since their problems are not real—but they're very real to them—that they have been exposed to some kind of unknown agent or whatever with perhaps unknown long-term effects that scare them very much. And people are saying to them your problems are not real.

More recently, a number of veterans and active duty military personnel have come forward with accounts of suspected chemical exposures that were confirmed, on-site, with the equipment that they had been trained with. They report how they were told then, and they are still being told, this was not real.

While we still have not been able to uncover the smoking gun—the smoking guns—responsible for these illnesses and health problems, research conducted by those outside the DOD and the VA, at the Centers for Disease Control, has shown that troops deployed to the Gulf were in fact three times as likely as troops who were deployed elsewhere in the Gulf to suffer fatigue, skin rashes, joint pain, headaches, diarrhea, and a long list of other things. Yet some continue to insist that because these serious health problems did not require lengthy hospitalizations, or they did not end up in death, that somehow they are not worthy of attention. I continue to vehemently reject that type of thinking, still bent on proving that we have no problem.

We have not done right by our veterans, after they have put themselves at enormous risk to protect our country, as they always do. That is my absolute belief. It is no surprise that they view the DOD, in the first instance, and less so the VA, with so little credibility because we can, and we must, do better.

Mr. Chairman, I know that you're aware that it is the Department of Defense, which, incidentally, is not appearing before us today, that continues to have primary responsibility for this issue. I've made it clear that in my view, DOD has not upheld their promise to provide adequate protection for the men and women who volunteered to go on this mission overseas which carried the clear—and soon to be present—danger of potential chemical weapons exposure. As I've often said, this was not Pearl Harbor. There was a long period of negotiation, then there was a long, systematic, logical, rational, slow, careful, methodical period of buildup where all kinds of things that could have been done by DOD were not done, to test and prepare for what might have been upcoming and, indeed, in some measure was upcoming.

It now appears that a new and invigorated, and perhaps even less biased, approach to the DOD investigation may be taking hold. Let's hope.

But I remain, Mr. Chairman, very concerned that the years of poor response by the Pentagon to the problems of these men and women has irrevocably undermined the public's faith in the ability of this Government to deal honestly with this issue. I regret that, and I think you and I seek to change that.

The credibility of DOD, as you pointed out, has suffered greatly not only because of this, but also because of other historical and current events, such as the problem of radiation experiments in the 1950's, Agent Orange in the 1970's, and allegations of sexual crimes and harassment against female military personnel in the 1990's. I realize there have been recent announcements and developments within DOD to try to remedy this. I hope that there will be clear opportunity to convince me and others that the approach has indeed changed at DOD.

I look forward to working with you, Mr. Chairman, on exploring ways of putting in place institutional safeguards, not only to find out what happened in this past 100 days war and afterwards, but to make sure that this kind of thing never happens again. We're worrying about our soldiers, men and women, this time, and we're worrying about our soldiers in all future wars which are likely to be fought on the same type of basis with chemicals and toxins in the future. No more Agent Oranges, no more Aberdeen Proving Grounds, please.

I have many concerns and questions about the Government's handling of these illnesses. They include, among others, why has VA denied almost 95 percent of the compensation claims for undiagnosed illnesses among Gulf War veterans, very often based upon what appears to me an arbitrary two-year time limit, which the Secretary is changing? Why have years of VA and DOD research investigating possible causes of the Gulf War illnesses proceeded without any attention to the possible chronic effects of exposures to low levels of nerve agents? Why did the DOD and the CIA insist that there was no possibility of exposures to chemical agents in the Gulf despite the existence of a 1991 CIA report describing the U.S. demolition of chemical munitions at Khamisiyah? Why did the intelligence community, CIA, and DOD fail to deal with the information on Khamisiyah and other possible exposures at the time that they occurred, not when they were forced into disclosure?

How could this happen in America? Was this due to some type of macho interagency rivalry, or simply poor communication? Or was it in fact something worse—a coverup?

Why is it that on one day this week we hear from the President's Advisory Committee that there is simply not enough evidence to support any cause of Persian Gulf War illness other than stress, but on the very next day we get word that independent, peer-reviewed but nongovernment research at the University of Texas again gives strong support to the possible linkage of drugs and pesticide and chemical exposures to these illnesses?

Well, I'll yield on that, Mr. Chairman. I will say, however, that it is simply outrageous that one individual Senator has stopped America's ratification of the Chemical Weapons Convention Treaty which would ban the development, production, possession, or transfer of chemical weapons on a worldwide basis—it would not solve the chemical problem, but it would certainly move towards that. This treaty has the support of the entire civilized world and would provide critical and immediate protection for our troops. There are lots of questions, with answers yet forthcoming. On the other hand, this issue is certainly in focus. I thank the Chairman.

[The opening statement of Senator Rockefeller appears on page 55.]

Chairman SPECTER. Thank you very much, Senator Rockefeller. The reference to the disclosures yesterday by a group of scientists headed by Dr. Robert Haley will be a matter of inquiry by this Committee. I had a chance to talk briefly to Dr. Haley yesterday by telephone. And without getting into the details as to his conclusions, there is some indication of the conclusion of exposure to chemical warfare as the source of the problems on a variety of symptoms of Gulf War Syndrome. We will be getting into that in some detail.

We turn now to the distinguished Secretary of Veterans Affairs, the Honorable Jesse Brown. Secretary Brown is a combat disabled Vietnam veteran. He enlisted in the Marine Corps in 1963. While in combat in 1965, he sustained gunshot wounds leaving his right arm partially paralyzed. He has had a distinguished record with the Disabled American Veterans, and he has served now as Secretary of Veterans Affairs for 4 years this month.

Secretary Brown is accompanied by Dr. Kenneth Kizer and Mr. Stephen Lemons.

To the extent possible, Secretary Brown, we would like you to limit your comments to the 5 to 10 minute range. We'll set the clock at 10 minutes. We're going to use 5 minute rounds for the Senators. But to the extent you can summarize your testimony, we would appreciate it, leaving the maximum time for dialogue, questions, and answers.

Welcome, and the floor is yours, Mr. Secretary.

STATEMENT OF HON. JESSE BROWN, SECRETARY OF VETERANS AFFAIRS; ACCOMPANIED BY HON. KENNETH KIZER, M.D., M.P.H., UNDER SECRETARY FOR HEALTH;

STEPHEN L. LEMONS, ACTING UNDER SECRETARY FOR BENEFITS

Secretary BROWN. Thank you so much, Mr. Chairman. I want to take advantage of this opportunity to congratulate you as you take over the Chair of this Committee. Your sensitivity to all veterans and your advocacy for those who have served in the Persian Gulf are well, well known. Of course, it is always good to see my good friend Senator Rockefeller, who has been a powerful supporter of our veterans and their families. And to my good friend Mr. Hutchinson, I'm glad to see that you decided to bring your dedication and your commitment from the House to the Senate. And to a real strong and compassionate fighter for veterans, Senator Wellstone.

Clearly, we face many challenges in pursuing our mutual goal of serving veterans and their families. Some issues, such as Persian Gulf Veterans' illnesses, are very, very complex. That is why I'm so pleased that this Committee will have knowledgeable and effective leadership during the 105th Congress.

With that, Mr. Chairman, let me thank you and the members of the Committee for the opportunity to discuss how VA is responding to the needs of Persian Gulf veterans. My prepared statement and other reports provided to the Committee fully describe what we have done and what we are doing. At this time, I will summarize this information including our response to low level exposure to chemical warfare agents.

To put this information into perspective, we recall that the media reports glamorized the war as 40 days and nights of thunder in the air and 100 hours of lightening on the ground. The rest of the story was not so appealing. Nearly 700,000 U.S. troops spent several months in a harsh desert environment. Our warriors were exposed to months of preparation for war with deep concerns about land mines, chemical and biological warfare attacks, and a well-armed enemy. They faced stressful combat conditions, smoke from oil fires, infectious parasites, drugs to counter the effects of nerve gas, insecticides, toxic petroleum products, and chemical agents.

When victory was declared, some of our servicemen and women found that their war was not over. Soon after returning from the war, veterans began to report a variety of illnesses and symptoms. They were suffering from fatigue, memory loss, painful joints, and other physical and psychological problems. We in the veterans community remembered the frustrations of Vietnam veterans waiting for a response to concerns about Agent Orange and we were determined that history should not repeat itself.

When I became Secretary for Veterans Affairs in January 1993, VA had already established a Persian Gulf registry. This was good. But we immediately strengthened it. We made this issue one of VA's top priorities. We requested and received legislation to give Persian Gulf veterans special eligibility for VA medical care. VA established four Persian Gulf referral centers. We named an expert scientific advisory committee with representatives from our veterans service organizations on it. We started an extensive research program including three environmental hazards research centers. We conducted nationwide clinical training for the staff caring for our Persian Gulf veterans. We consolidated Persian Gulf benefits claims to ensure consistency and fair ratings. And we supported legislation to compensate Persian Gulf veterans with undiagnosed illnesses.

As you know, Mr. Chairman, this law states that veterans must have symptoms within a presumptive period, now established at 2 years after they left the Persian Gulf. I am very concerned that some of the claims were denied because their symptoms did not appear until after the 2-year presumptive period. I wrote to the President to propose that the current presumptive period be reconsidered. I am pleased that earlier this week the President announced that he has accepted my proposal, and I am charged with reporting back to him in 60 days regarding extending the limit. I want you to know, sir, that I will consult with the veterans organizations, Members of Congress, and other interested parties before making my decision.

When the compensation law was passed we initiated an aggressive outreach program to inform Persian Gulf veterans. We immediately began reviewing environmental hazard claims that had been denied. We all know that health-related problems associated with the Persian Gulf can only be answered through research. The President has designated me to take the lead in coordinating all federally sponsored research. More than 80 Persian Gulf research projects are now in progress and others have been completed. Large VA studies include a long-term mortality study of Persian Gulf veterans and a national health survey of those veterans and their families. Last year, VA established a fourth environmental hazard research center to study the possibility of reproductive problems related to military service. We are proud that nearly half of all Persian Gulf research is being conducted at VA hospitals and our affiliated medical schools. But it is also important, sir, to work with independent and nongovernment experts, and that is why we have worked closely with the Persian Gulf expert scientific panel, the National Academy of Sciences' Institute of Medicine, the National Institutes of Health, and the American Institute for Biological Sciences. And that is also why we have supported research by nongovernment scientists.

Following DOD's announcement in June 1996 that U.S. troops may have been exposed to chemical warfare agents in the Persian Gulf, we moved aggressively to evaluate this information. The available scientific literature suggests that long-term chronic health problems do not result from exposures that were not marked by acute clinical science and symptoms. However, research in this area is clearly limited. We cannot conclude that low level exposures do not have long-term effects, especially when combined with other environmental factors. More research is needed. Accordingly, the Persian Gulf Veterans Coordinating Board requested, and received, funding for three research projects to study low level exposure to chemicals.

Mr. Chairman, we are, and have been, very proactive on the problems reported by Persian Gulf veterans. We are examining Persian Gulf veterans; 62,000 have completed registry examinations, and all who have reported symptoms have been treated seriously and received appropriate medical evaluations. We are treating Persian Gulf veterans—187,000 outpatient visits, 19,000 hospital stays, and 74,000 counseled at Vet Centers. We're working to compensate Persian Gulf veterans. We wrote to 44,000 Persian Gulf veterans and invited them to file claims. We are reviewing 11,000 cases to make sure that they were developed and adjudicated properly. And we continue to search for answers.

I have said on many occasions that if anyone believes we should be doing something that we're not doing, we want to hear from you. That is why I was surprised, quite frankly, at some of the criticism that I've heard. It has been suggested, for example, that the VA did not listen to veterans who said that they were exposed to chemical warfare agents in the Persian Gulf. The record shows that VA acted responsibly and aggressively even while DOD said there were no significant exposures. In 1993, for instance, VA designed a special clinical protocol that was meant to detect symptoms related to nerve gas exposures. On November 1, 1993, we responded to a group of veterans who said they had been exposed to chemical warfare agents. We selected the Birmingham VA Medical Center to investigate their concerns. The research center developed a specialized neurological examination to look into the effects of chemical agents. This facility continues to serve as a focal point for referral patients including those with chemical agents exposures. On November 16, 1993, I said before this Committee our search for answers has never ruled out chemical agents. And in the spring of 1994, we revised a registry questionnaire and code sheet to ask veterans if they believed they were exposed to chemical agents. These efforts continue to be important and they are being carried out every day in VA facilities across the Nation.

I believe that most VA employees feel, as I do, that Persian Gulf veterans are not faceless statistics. They are individual Americans who answered their country's call and served bravely. They are individuals who come to us with real problems and concerns about their future. We are absolutely committed to responding to those problems and concerns with efficiency and compassion.

Mr. Chairman, this concludes my statement. I will be happy to respond to any questions that you or members of this Committee may have.

[The prepared statement of Mr. Brown appears on page 62.]

Chairman SPECTER. Thank you very much, Secretary Brown.

We will have 5-minute rounds for the members to question.

Mr. Secretary, on the issue of a 2-year presumption so that if symptoms are not reported within 2 years there's no response by the Veterans Administration, it seems to me surprising that would be a rule. There are many ailments which take a very long time to manifest themselves. Asbestos, illustratively, comes up after a decade or a decade and a half. Many symptoms are not known within a short period like two years. Do you have the authority yourself to expand that two year presumptive period?

Secretary BROWN. Yes, sir, I do.

Chairman SPECTER. Well, why don't you do it today?

Secretary BROWN. Because I want to consult with the veterans organizations, the Members of Congress, and other interested groups to determine what would be an appropriate extension. We're dealing with something that we do not have any scientific experience with. You mentioned asbestos, I could mention a number of others that we have in the presumptive period, such as multiple sclerosis—

Chairman SPECTER. Well, why not extend it beyond two years effective immediately with a determination at a later date as to how long the period is extended to?

Secretary BROWN. I already have an agreement with the President that I will investigate this and I will get back with him in 60 days with a recommendation on the extension. That is what we plan on doing.

Chairman SPECTER. Mr. Secretary, with all due respect, I don't think that's adequate. I've been talking to a lot of veterans myself in my own State, in Allentown, in Pittsburgh, in Philadelphia, and there is enormous concern and it manifests itself at a number of levels. One is, as to whether they're getting the adequate medical care they need. But so many others are saying we just want to be treated fairly.

Now, the veterans groups are not going to tell you not to extend it, the Congress is not going to tell you not to extend it. Senator Rockefeller and I believe we could enact legislation this month, certainly early next month, to extend the period of time. I think it would be a very salutary thing if in your capacity as Secretary of Veterans Affairs you said here and now the period is extended, we'll determine what the cutoff date is, whether it's three years, four years, five years, or ten years. But let the word go out today to the veterans of American that action is being taken now, that there is no longer a two year period, that it is extended and we'll tell you at a later time how long it is extended to. Why not?

Secretary BROWN. I don't believe that is really the way to develop public policy. I think that there needs to be a structure by which we obtain justification for extending it. I have to tell you another reason why I am in favor of extending it, I received a letter from Senator Wellstone expressing his concern about this some time ago.

What we want to do is make sure that we're doing the right thing by our veterans. We're going to evaluate all of the data that we have. We're going to have public forums all around the country, there will be at least six of them, where we talk directly to the veterans on how they feel and how we should go about resolving this matter. And I will be consulting with our veterans organizations here in Washington. So we're going to do the right thing, sir. I believe that the veterans community will be very happy and responsive to the conclusion that we reach.

Chairman SPECTER. Mr. Secretary, I respectfully disagree. I don't think there's any doubt anywhere that that presumption limit to two years is unfair and medically inaccurate. I urge you to give consideration to extending that period today. I think it would be a bold, necessary, important step forward if the Secretary of Veterans Affairs said today that two year presumptive period is no longer in effect. Listen, there are veterans going to hospitals all across America today who are being told their complaints are too late. In the time that it is going to take for the review, 60 days, there will be thousands of veterans who will be turned away. There is no doubt that it is going to be extended. The only issue to be decided is for how long.

While you were giving your last response, Senator Rockefeller leaned over and whispered to me—that goes to show you the level of cooperation—that I have his support. Think about it during the course of the hearing. I think it would be a really important signal if that were done today, Mr. Secretary. Think it over in the course of the morning's hearing.

Mr. Secretary, let me proceed to the issue of all of the competing, conflicting medical evidence which we have on the subject. You have listed a great many boards and agencies which are considering the issue as to the cause of these ailments. What I would like to do, and perhaps this question ought to be addressed to Dr. Kizer, I would like to have in the VA a focal point starting now to review and analyze all of the evidence which is available, and to have our staff work with you immediately to try to collate that evidence and to try to bring it to a conclusion and not to wait until we have a further hearing, which will be down the road in a matter of the next few weeks, but to try to come to a conclusion now and make a medical determination as to the sufficiency of the existing studies and whether anything additionally needs to be done on those studies.

Dr. Kizer, how could that be structured medically and scientifically?

Dr. KIZER. The issue is actually resolved. We do not have all the answers. We have ongoing review of the data. It is clear by the number of research studies that there are many things that are not answered. We are continually reviewing the data. As new studies come out, there is going to continue to arise questions that further research is going to need to clarify.

Chairman SPECTER. We have a great many at least tentative answers. When I go through the evidence, I am unable to digest it all because I'm not a trained scientist or a trained physician or an expert in the these lines. I would like to have one focal point, an expert. The Veterans Administration is the most logical place for it, it seems to me, to take all the studies and line them all up, including the one by Dr. Haley and the ones from the presidential commission. We may need technical assistance from you or Mr. Secretary, or we may turn to Secretary Shalala of Health and Human Services, or we may go out and hire our own. I don't think we need to reinvent the wheel; we have the existing expertise. But I would like to see a hard line collation of all of the studies we have now with what conclusions we have, and an articulation of what the unanswered questions are so that we can focus on those. It may be that you will need some assistance legislatively on the subject.

I would like you to direct your attention to that kind of a collation so that we could get an answer to precisely what we know, precisely what the studies have shown, and precisely what we yet have to inquire into. Would you help us on that, Mr. Secretary?

Secretary BROWN. Absolutely. I have no problem in making a commitment that we will help you to pull together all of the existing literature, try to determine exactly what it means, and where we need to go from there.

Chairman SPECTER. Thank you very much. My time expired during the course of the last question. I yield now to Senator Rockefeller.

Senator ROCKEFELLER. Thank you, Mr. Chairman.

Secretary Brown, first of all, let's put it in the record—you have fought hard for veterans, there is no question about that, on this and all other matters. You have been hindered by people not being forthcoming with a lot of information which has been, therefore, not available to you. I think one of the things that Chairman Specter has in mind is that you may have rulemaking and public comment problems in your so-called 60 days or whatever, and that the Congress can do it without that. We can simply pass a law—I think it could pass very easily, without some of the administrative or rulemaking problems that you might have. I know that you want to do it and I know you convinced the President to do it. He announced yesterday that he wanted to do it. But I think that Chairman Specter is right, we should do it as fast as possible.

Secretary BROWN. Senator Rockefeller, if the Congress wishes to resolve this, I have no objection whatsoever.

Senator ROCKEFELLER. And I knew you wouldn't. I knew that.

Dr. Kizer, this is a question for you, sir. First of all, there isn't any thought in your head that this is simply a matter of stress and psychological worries on the part of these harmed Persian Gulf veterans, is there? You're not of that school?

Dr. KIZER. I'm not sure what you're asking, sir.

Senator ROCKEFELLER. In other words, the other answer expressed is that PB and low level chemical agents and other types of things have no deep effect on any of this?

Dr. KIZER. Let me answer you in part by asking a question, because your question, while it was very simple at face value, is not at all simple. Last month a very good study in the Journal Circulation was published that showed that people with depression have a four times higher rate of heart attack than those without. Does that mean that their heart attacks are not real?

Senator ROCKEFELLER. No, don't play games with me, please.

Dr. KIZER. I'm not playing games.

Senator ROCKEFELLER. I asked you a question, and that is, you do agree, don't you, that this is more complicated than simply a matter of something called "stress."

Dr. KIZER. I think our Persian Gulf veterans have illnesses, and they need to be treated. Now, what etiologic role stress may play in some cases I think is a matter of ongoing investigation.

Senator ROCKEFELLER. So, there is a hint that you may be of that school. You don't have a presumption?

Dr. KIZER. I think you are over-simplifying the connection between the mind and the body.

Senator ROCKEFELLER. I am over-simplifying because I'm worried about your presumption.

Dr. KIZER. When somebody experience a stressful event and they develop Grave's disease, that disease is very real even though it may have been precipitated by stress. When someone develops diabetes because of a stressful event, their diabetes is very real even though it may have been precipitated by a stressful event. So I don't think it is as straightforward as you imply.

Senator ROCKEFELLER. I know that. I am also more worried now about your answer than I was before. Be that as it may, the chairwoman of VA's own Persian Gulf expert scientific committee, Dr. Bingham, who is a highly respected toxicologist, recently said that Persian Gulf veterans were clearly experiencing more health problems than any other veterans. She also said that it is much too early to rule out drugs, pyridostigmine bromide being one of those, and the effect of pyridostigmine bromide when mixed with DEET—which Dr. Moss was working on and then was fired and still has not a job—that, and chemical agents, and other factors. It's much too early to rule these things out as a cause of the problems, she said. And most importantly, she said it is much too early to point to stress as the only remaining cause. She said that. In fact, she complained that those who are now primarily pointing to stress haven't even studied it scientifically as a possibility, that they sort of fall back on that, not having other things to put forward which are declarative.

So, what would you have us believe about this?

Dr. KIZER. As you know from my testimony before you, as well as my testimony before Mr. Specter last December, I am very much in agreement with those comments. We are keeping a very open mind to all of those things. I don't think you're saying anything that is at all at variance to the position that the VA has.

Senator ROCKEFELLER. All right. Secretary Brown and Dr. Kizer, you obviously know about the articles on the Persian Gulf War illnesses that will appear in next week's JAMA, Journal of the American Medical Association. One of them is a study of Iowa Persian Gulf veterans that was conducted by the Centers for Disease Control, and there are also three studies by Dr. Haley and some of his associates at the University of Texas Southwestern Medical Center that Chairman Specter referred to. These studies contribute to the accumulating research that indicates that a significant percentage of the Gulf War veterans have chronic and serious health problems which they attribute to their time in the Gulf. Two of these studies also suggested additional evidence of "delayed, chronic, neurotoxic syndromes" which may well be related to the combination of environmental exposures to agents such as pyridostigmine bromide, insecticides, exposures to low level chemicals, et cetera.

What is your reaction to these findings? How do they compare to the reports of VA-funded research and the Persian Gulf War Registry?

Dr. KIZER. As you note, the studies will be published in next week's issue. We have just been able to obtain a copy of them and are looking at those studies in detail. The results from Iowa are very similar to the study that we requested of the veterans in Pennsylvania as far as self-reported symptoms among those veterans. So they seem to be very similar in results.

As far as Dr. Haley's studies, those are something that need to be looked at in detail. The one thing that is certainly notable about them is that they involve a very small sample size. That is something that has to be looked at as far as how far those findings, looking at 23 patients, can be extrapolated to a larger universe, particularly with some of the statistical methodology that was used. All I am saying is that we need to look at it. We're in the process of doing that, and we will be following up on it. They are similar in content to a number of studies that the VA is also conducting.

Senator ROCKEFELLER. Yes. Mr. Chairman, I just have to notice, although I'm running over my time here, that Dr. Abou-Donia, Dr. Moss, the early University of Texas studies—there's a lot of people who say there is a growing body of independent, peer-reviewed research—peer-reviewed—that continues to find evidence of just such a linkage. You're not being very specific about it; others are being specific. In other words, drugs, chemical hazards, other problems, a combination of things. I worry about this and I worry about people's refusal to be more forthcoming about it. I thank the Chairman.

Chairman SPECTER. Senator Rockefeller, I share that view and that concern. That's why the first issue that I raised with the Secretary was getting the expertise out of the Veterans Administration, perhaps out of HHS, or wherever so that we take a look at it all, that before coming back to the glare of the hearing room, we sit down and try to put the pieces together in a puzzle around a table in my office or yours. We really get down to brass tacks and take a look at all the medical evidence which is around, and maybe even bring the doctors in in an informal session in which we can get more out factually than we do here. But we've got to come to grips with it. There is a lot of evidence, as Senator Rockefeller says, about causal connection. We've got to pinpoint it and not just let it drag out from one hearing to another. We intend to do that.

Dr. KIZER. Mr. Chairman, if I might just respond a little bit. I may not have been as clear as perhaps I should have been in earlier response to you. But what you're asking is something, and what I intended to say, is something that is being done. The research working group does that. The research group is composed of representatives from HHS and from VA as well as from DOD. Likewise, the Institute of Medicine has done that and has published their reviews. They have an ongoing function in this regard.

So, the task or the objective that you are asking for is something that is being done. We'll be more than happy to sit down with you or others and talk about where it is at this point in time.

Senator ROCKEFELLER. On our next round, Mr. Chairman, I definitely have a question for Dr. Kizer on that.

Chairman SPECTER. Senator Rockefeller, I don't think there is going to be another round unless we're going to be here until tomorrow. So if you have another question, you're ranking, take another moment or two.

Senator ROCKEFELLER. Let me just ask this. The early VA research and clinical evaluations of Persian Gulf War illnesses did not assess for possible exposures or look at possible chronic effects of low level chemical agents or organophosphates. And that was for a very good reason. DOD insisted that there was no such thing and no such possibility that our troops had been exposed to chemical weapons. We now know that to be totally without basis. But you had to go ahead and conduct research based upon what you were hearing at the time from them.

Those revelations have since come out. We now know differently. Therefore, I think it is fair to ask, what action has VA undertaken to change its research agenda based upon this new knowledge that there was more involved? I want you to be specific, Dr. Kizer; what new studies have been funded? How many? Exactly what is being studied? What specific changes have been made in the ongoing studies and registries?

Dr. KIZER. I think I would as a preface to that just clarify that even though the DOD insisted that there was no chemical exposure, the Department has been open to that possibility. Senator Hutchinson probably recalls chastising me, and chastising may be a little bit too strong, at a hearing a couple of years ago for statements that I made in the press challenging that supposition.

Our Registry exam has had throughout the process questions related to this, as have our clinical protocols. So we have absolutely remained open to this possibility. Of course, the most difficult thing in this regard from a clinical perspective is that there simply is no scientific test, no diagnostic test, to test for the specific effects of a chemical warfare agent exposure.

As far as what has happened since the revelations, if you will, of the Khamisiyah incident, VA has conducted a number of things as far as education for our clinical personnel. We are developing a specific research strategy, a broad strategy in this regard. Three studies have been funded for this. There is a Request For Proposal that is out on the street. Proposals need to be submitted by February 19. After those proposals have been reviewed, then there will be a longer list of studies that have been funded. As I have testified before Mr. Specter, as well as yourself, we believe the research agenda in this regard has been delayed because of the belief that there was no exposure in this regard.

Senator ROCKEFELLER. I am told that there is $2.5 million that is under negotiation for research, about $2 million of proposals for research, but that nothing is ongoing in the way of research.

Dr. KIZER. As I understand it, three studies have been funded for about $2.2 million; and the Request For Proposals that is out on the street is for $2.5 million, and then there's another $9-plus million for proposals that are also to be submitted by the February date that I mentioned.

Senator ROCKEFELLER. We'll find out more about that. Thank you, Mr. Chairman.

Chairman SPECTER. Dr. Kizer, when those matters are pursued, the Committee would like the unconventional views incorporated as well. Dr. Moss, Dr. Nicholson, Dr. Baumsweiger, wherever the views are coming from, we would like to have them reviewed and commented on.

Senator Hutchinson, we welcome you to the Senate and to this Committee. This is your maiden line of questioning. The floor is yours.

Senator HUTCHINSON. Thank you, Mr. Chairman. Let me first of all extend my congratulations on your election to the Chairmanship of the Committee. I look forward to working with you. I am delighted personally to be able to come over from the House and, serving on the Veterans Affairs' Committee on the House side, be able to continue my interest in veterans' issues, my support for veterans by serving on your Committee in the Senate. So I congratulate you. I will be drawing on my House experience and certainly public concern for the health and well-being of over 700,000 men and women who served during the Gulf War. And for those who continue to serve in East Asia, the concern for these continues to mount with each new revelation by the Pentagon and other sources on chemical exposures to U.S. ground personnel during the war.

The veterans of the Persian Gulf War deserve in expeditious fashion to be dealt with truthfully in all aspects of their service. Frankly, it is unconscionable to me that the Federal Government has been less than forthcoming in the information provided to these veterans and the American public.

Dr. Kizer, I suspect I should have been more skeptical during the hearings that we had on the House side in which the Department of Defense repeatedly assured us of no chemical exposure in the Gulf War theater. Richard Cohen wrote in the Washington Post day before yesterday, "From the outset, they"—and that means the veterans, and that means the Veterans' Affairs Committee, and that means the veteran service organizations and everybody else—"they were told that reports of chemical weapons use were wholly imaginary, sheerest rumor, unsubstantiated twaddle, a lie, or a damned lie depending upon who the briefing officer was at the time." That's what we all heard and we heard it over and over again. That's what you heard, Mr. Secretary.

Mr. Cohen then poses this issue, and I think it is quite legitimate, has anyone in the military been fired, demoted, punished, or even chastised for insisting against mounting evidence to the contrary that no American troops were exposed to chemical or biological agents during or after the Gulf War. That issue is totally apart and separate from what Senator Rockefeller was addressing as to the causal relationship and whether or not it is the cause of the symptoms that veterans have detected and expressed. But it is a very important issue. I know it is not appropriate today, we don't have the DOD officials here, but that I think deserves answers as to why it happened and whether anything has been done by way of punishment of those. The Pentagon is not just a building; it's people. Somewhere that misinformation originated.

Mr. Secretary, I just want to pick up on the plan to extend the two year period. I understand the President supports changing the disability rules, apparently everybody supports changing the disability rules, to change the two year period that has been in place in the past. I had a veteran in Rodgers, Arkansas, back in my home State, who had been contacted by the VA and asked to come in and have a physical to determine whether or not he had any of these symptoms. Well, he hadn't had any of these symptoms, had no complaints. But then a little seed was planted, well, maybe, maybe I'm entitled to something, and he'll be going in. I am just wondering, is it going to be three years, four years, five years, how far do we liberalize that policy?

Secretary BROWN. Senator Hutchinson, that's one of the reasons why it is so very important that I talk with the veterans groups, that I talk with Members of Congress, that I talk with our scientists, our adjudication people to get a sense of exactly how far we should extend that presumptive period. There has to be a rational basis for the extension.

Senator HUTCHINSON. Under a liberalized policy, is it conceivable that the VA would bear the responsibility of compensating all 700,000 who served for illnesses that may not be connected to their service? We're talking about undiagnosed, as you pointed out.

Secretary BROWN. You're absolutely correct. And that's the problem. Historically, particularly as you know, all of our presumptive periods have been based on science or there has been a scientific relationship between a disease occurring concurrent with active duty and manifesting itself 1, 2, or 7 years out into the future. The conditions that we're dealing with, with respect to the Persian Gulf, we don't know very much about them. That's what all of this science is about. But at the same time, we know our veterans are sick. So we want to have a mechanism that responds to them until we're able to allow the science to catch up so, hopefully, we'll be able to cure them.

Senator HUTCHINSON. That's exactly the goal of Congress in what we've implemented in going ahead and providing that health care to them.

Secretary BROWN. Well, for the first time in the VA's history, we have never before compensated veterans for undiagnosed illnesses. They really can be defined as things like headaches, painful joints, memory loss. These are more symptoms—

Senator HUTCHINSON. Mr. Secretary, that light is going to go off and I have to ask one more question. I have been waiting too long and there is not going to be another round.

Chairman SPECTER. One more question, Senator Hutchinson.

Senator HUTCHINSON. Thank you. Dr. Kizer, with not knowing how far we liberalize it, responsibly implementing a liberalization program on that two years, how would we expand that? How would that affect the budget? Are there any estimates on the budget impact? And will we be denying other veterans proper health care because of the budget constraints under a liberalized policy?

Secretary BROWN. Senator Hutchinson, I think I have to answer that one. First of all, I have a basic philosophy that we shouldn't be taking money from one group of veterans to fund another group of veterans. Anytime you put Americans at risk and they come home suffering from all kinds of diseases and injuries, we shouldn't be asking ourselves how we're going to pay to create a level playing field. So that's one of the reasons why we have to move forward with reasonableness, and that's what we're going to do. We've established a timetable here of 60 days. Now, on the other hand, if the Congress said we want to do it tomorrow, I support them 100 percent. But we want to move forward to look at everything to make sure that we protect our Persian Gulf veterans while at the same time we make sure that we do not place at risk another group of veterans in order to achieve the initial goal.

Senator HUTCHINSON. Thank you, Mr. Secretary. Thank you, Mr. Chairman.

Chairman SPECTER. Thank you, Senator Hutchinson. Senator Wellstone.

Senator WELLSTONE. Thank you, Mr. Chairman. First of all, Mr. Chairman, for the record, I listened carefully to some of the questions you put to the Secretary which I think were absolutely appropriate. I appreciate your tenacious advocacy. Back in late December, after having met with Gulf veterans and just being very moved by men and women who, and I'm quoting directly, were "scared to death" because they just didn't know what was happening to them, I sent a letter saying at least we ought to extend this presumptive period. So I really appreciate this. I think I suggested 10 years. But I think we have to know. Maybe it will be indefinitely.

One thing I did want to say is to put in a kind word about Secretary Brown's advocacy for veterans. I think the real good news is that whether or not the Secretary today declares a specific length of time we're going to see an extension. If I go back to the last Congress and some of the battles that we had when it came to cuts in benefits for veterans, the veterans community is well aware of the fact that this Secretary of Veterans Affairs was out there for veterans. So, Secretary Brown says that he is committed to making sure that something is done about this presumptive period. What we've had now is a lot of people being denied claims. I don't think, Senator Hutchinson, that—altogether there have been about 11,000 or so claims made and we had about 697,000 veterans there—I don't think we're going to ever have to worry about veterans all of a sudden stepping forward and saying they were ill or sick if they're not struggling with these illnesses. Veterans won't do that. In fact, a lot of veterans I've talked to were embarrassed about having to go public at all. But the point is that a lot of people did get turned down and some of them because it was outside that two year window. But when Secretary Brown says that he is committed to being out there and he is committed to extending this—and maybe we'll do it legislatively, fine—I don't think there is any question about his word. I don't think there is any question at all in the veterans community about his word on this. It will be done.

After having said that just for the record, I wanted to just go back to two questions. This is one that I think Senator Rockefeller was going to ask and it is a question that just has come to my attention. In looking at the VA statistical records on Gulf veterans—and maybe this is for Dr. Kizer—my understanding, and it may be wrong, is that one possible problem is that potentially there were a lot of veterans, thousands of veterans who chose to go to private hospitals so that they weren't actually a part of the database that you had, which of course could have really skewed your findings. Isn't that a problem in terms of your assessment of where we're now?

My second question for any of you is could you give us some assessment of the kind of care people are getting, given that we don't know exactly why they're struggling with these different illnesses? And I feel that in Minnesota people are getting good care, that's what I'm hearing, as good care as they can get given the fact that we don't know the source of the problem.

And then my third point, and it is not a question, is that I have this idea that could be wrong, I'm a lay person, I'm not a scientist, but the Texas research that is going to be coming out in JAMA, is going to address talking about multiple chemical exposure, right? Talking about what happens with the interaction of multiple chemicals. Well, let me tell you, this has got incredible implications. Chemical companies are going to be very interested in this and so should all of us be as consumers. We don't do that kind of testing of interactions between chemicals and pesticides. All sorts of different agencies don't do that when they look at the potential harm for people. We should be doing that. This has tremendous implications. I'm glad they've done the research. I'm glad JAMA is publishing it. I have a feeling though that even after that's done and even after the Chairman and others do everything they can to get to the bottom of this, the evidence is still going to be ambiguous within the scientific community. So then the policy question becomes, what do we do when we're not certain? And it seems to me we should err on the side of veterans. It then becomes simple. We should make sure they get the care and they get the compensation.

Two questions there. Just your response, then I'm done.

Chairman SPECTER. Is there a question pending?

Senator WELLSTONE. I already put the question. You were gone while the question was asked.

Chairman SPECTER. I was listening. I heard the loudspeaker. I didn't hear a question, but if Dr. Kizer did, respond.

Dr. KIZER. There were multiple questions with multiple parts.

Senator WELLSTONE. Multiple questions.

Chairman SPECTER. Choose any two you like. [Laughter.]

Senator WELLSTONE. You stay out of this, Mr. Chairman. [Laughter.]

Chairman SPECTER. Oh, no, I'm not going to stay out of this. I'm the Chairman. [Laughter.]

Dr. KIZER. Senator Wellstone asked a question which segues very nicely with what Senator Hutchinson asked as well. The question about the presumptive period here really applies to the compensation. Medical care is being provided already.

Senator WELLSTONE. That's right.

Dr. KIZER. There is no time limit on the medical care. The medical care that is being provided is basically tailored to what the patient needs. If they have minimal complaints, they are evaluated and we try to address it. The overwhelming majority of patients who have been seen have diagnoses and are receiving treatment. There is a significant number, though, that have not been diagnosed, and they are receiving symptomatic treatment as best as possible. Not surprisingly, and similar to what we see in the academic world and elsewhere, when you're not able to diagnose somebody and not able to tell them what's wrong with them, they often aren't as satisfied with their care and they go around to multiple different providers trying to find an answer. That's not unique to Gulf War veterans by any means.

Senator WELLSTONE. The question on your database was the other one.

Dr. KIZER. The database, because there has been such an open door policy as far as this, we don't think that is a big problem. It is something that we would certainly like for the sake of completeness, and we certainly request it when the veterans come in to get their records. There is variable compliance with that.

Chairman SPECTER. Thank you very much, Senator Wellstone. Senator Murray.

Senator MURRAY. Thank you, Mr. Chairman. I join my colleagues in welcoming you as Chair of this Committee and I look forward to working with you. I especially commend you for having this as one of the first hearings in this Congress to focus on the Gulf War Syndrome. I think it is very important that we send a message to veterans, both past veterans and future veterans, that this is an issue that we take very seriously. I think your having a hearing this soon sends that message, and I thank you.

Mr. Secretary, it is a delight to see you here. The veterans in my State wanted me to convey to you that they are pleased that you are going to continue your service to this country as you have for so many years. They send you their very best.

Secretary BROWN. Thank you.

Senator MURRAY. Mr. Chairman, everywhere I go in my State, small towns, large towns, Bellingham, Spokane, Vancouver, Seattle, vets come up to me and they are concerned about the Gulf War Syndrome. They ask the question that Senator Wellstone stated, which is, what is happening to me. I think it is absolutely essential that we find the answers to those questions quickly; otherwise, others will come up with answers for us and it will not do any of good in the long run. We need absolute openness on this condition, and I really urge all of us to continue in this direction.

My bottom line is for the vets who have served us and to make sure that they get the health care that they need quickly, in an efficient manner, and are taken care of. Mr. Secretary, I want to ask you if you believe that our vets are getting their health care needs met and that there is not any delay due to lack of information or the slow process of this.

Secretary BROWN. Senator Murray, I believe that we're doing the best that we can with what is known. The bottom line is that we simply do not know what we're dealing with. Take for instance a number of our veterans, not many, but a number of our Persian Gulf veterans with unexplained illnesses are coming to our facilities sick, and when we give them a complete workup we can't find any abnormalities. So we don't know what to treat. So they leave dissatisfied. What we are going to have to do is to continue to invest very heavily in research all across the board. Until we find out exactly what we're dealing with and then find some real solutions to this, we're not going to be able to craft a public policy to deal with this. The scientists are the ones who are going to have to help us out on trying to bring some quality of life back into the lives of our Persian Gulf veterans.

Senator MURRAY. And that concerns me when they leave dissatisfied. I understand that we can't answer every question they have, but it does arise to allowing other groups to provide them with answers. I specifically can tell you that in my State a group did hold an event, they spent more than $20,000 promoting it including radio and television advertisements and they mailed more than 100,000 invitations. Several hundred people attended and they were told that the Gulf War Syndrome was a communicable disease transmitted through perspiration, blood transfusion, and sexual contact. And if we don't find the answers, someone else out there is going to be giving them.

Secretary BROWN. One of the things I wasn't prepared to announce this morning, but if Dr. Murphy and Dr. Kizer allow me to tell you, we are aware of that and we're trying to set up counseling to our Persian Gulf veterans when they come in to explain everything that we know about it. If we are unable to help them, then we need to explain why we're not able to help them. And if they need further follow-up, we need to do that. We're going to have different types of mechanisms in place not only at the treating facility, but also at the VISN level. Dr. Kizer is working on that concept to allow us to get around the kinds of problems that you are describing which are very, very real.

Senator MURRAY. I appreciate that for that reason, because I also think we need to send a message to everyone that when people serve our country that we give them the health care that they need and we take care of it. So I appreciate that.

Let me ask you one other question, Mr. Secretary, in the short amount of time I have. I am concerned about this stress focus that's been placed because it does leave a lot of questions. Just your own personal view on the stress issue.

Secretary BROWN. First of all, it has always been my view that something is drastically wrong. When we first started looking at this in 1992–1993 people were saying to me that it's in their heads. We rejected that. We were looking, and we will continue to look for an organic basis. But at the same time, I really like what Dr. Lashof had to say about this. She is basically saying that we need to have a better understanding of the relationship between stress and physical disability. If a person because of stress has a heart attack, that heart attack is just as real to that individual as if it were induced by the arterial sclerotic process. So we need to understand that. It has implications not only for future warriors, but it also has implications all across our society. The relationship between stress and physical disability is a valid scientific question and we need to look at it, and we're going to do that in the VA.

Senator MURRAY. Thank you. Thank you, Mr. Chairman.

Chairman SPECTER. Thank you very much, Senator Murray.

Thank you very much, Secretary Brown, Dr. Kizer, and Dr. Lemons. This is a good start. We are going to be following up on this this afternoon. I've already instructed our staff director Charles Battaglia to be in contact with your department, Mr. Secretary, to pursue the issue of focusing in on the medical issues and a comparison as to what the various studies have found. I appreciate, as Dr. Kizer has said, that there has been that kind of analysis and review. We would like to take a look at it ourselves.

There is a real sense of urgency that we try to collate it and put it all together to find out what the underlying conclusions are, whether we have enough basis for conclusions. We can make legislative conclusions. Legislative conclusions may be just a little different than medical conclusions, but we can make legislative conclusions. If there are other studies that need to be undertaken, let us make that determination. You may need some legislative help on that and we're prepared to give that assistance.

Secretary Brown, I would like you to consider the issue of making the extension today. On reflecting on my request to you, maybe it would be something that you would want to consult with the President about since you have told him you would report to him within 60 days. That may be something that Senator Rockefeller and I will take up with the President as well so that you do not have an obligation to wait or give a 60 day period. Or we can move ahead on legislation. But there are many, many veterans who will be at veterans hospitals across America between now and March 8. So I would like you to give that some thought and perhaps consult with the White House on it.

Secretary BROWN. Thank you so much for your concern, sir.

Chairman SPECTER. We appreciate you very much, gentlemen. Thank you.

We now call our next panel. We have the Acting Director of Central Intelligence, George Tenet, and Executive Director of the Central

Intelligence Agency, Ms. Nora Slatkin, who will be sitting with Director Tenet.

We welcome you here, Director Tenet. You come before this Veterans' Committee as a good friend. You have a distinguished record having served on the National Security Council, having been staff director for the Senate Committee on Intelligence, and, on a personal level, if I may say, having known you for many years, from your service with my distinguished colleague, Senator John Heinz of Pennsylvania. I had alluded earlier to the finding of the President's commission and, in introducing you, I think it appropriate to read from page 37 of the final report: "CIA has systematically reviewed classified and open source information relating to chemical, biological warfare agent exposures during the Gulf War." And then in contrast, "Department of Defense has failed to take advantage of its unique access to both classified and routine military operations and intelligence records." So that contrast is very significant. You are joined also by Ms. Sylvia Copeland and we welcome her here. We look forward to your testimony. To the extent that you can summarize it, we would appreciate it.

STATEMENT OF GEORGE J. TENET, ACTING DIRECTOR OF CENTRAL INTELLIGENCE ACCOMPANIED BY NORA SLATKIN, EXECUTIVE DIRECTOR, CENTRAL INTELLIGENCE AGENCY; SYLVIA COPELAND, ANALYST, OFFICE OF STRATEGIC WEAPONS RESEARCH, CENTRAL INTELLIGENCE AGENCY

Mr. TENET. Thank you, Senator, for inviting us here today. This is an important issue for us and for you and we want to do everything that we can to help the Committee and our veterans get to the bottom of a difficult issue. I hope that I can also during my testimony answer some of the questions that Senator Rockefeller posed in his opening statement.

To go over the background first, the CIA has focused its energies on the intelligence aspects of this issue. We began a comprehensive review of all intelligence reporting in March of 1995. We started at this date because of the President's concerns and because of the issue raised by CIA employees. Until then we were focused on uncovering still hidden elements of Iraq's chemical and biological weapons program. This work was important to support UNSCOM's effort to eliminate these programs. In our review, we examined all the intelligence reporting to help DOD determine whether or not U.S. troops were exposed to chemical or biological agents during the Gulf War. The exposure could have been either through Iraqi use or through destruction of Iraq's chemical or biological facilities.

In 1995 we identified Khamisiyah, and I'll come back to Khamisiyah in depth, as a potential exposure site in the course of this effort. We then took the initiative to determine what happened there. The Presidential Advisory Committee last spring then asked us to arrange to model events during and after the war resulting in the release of chemical agents into the atmosphere.

As we told you during a briefing in September 1996, we used a contractor to model releases at Muhammadiyat, Al Muthanna, and Bunker 73 at Khamisiyah. We were unable to have the contractor model the pit area destruction at Khamisiyah in March of 1991. The data were simply too uncertain. After long efforts, we think that everything possible has been done to try to model the chemical release at the Khamisiyah pit. We have learned lessons from our work; we will draw on them in the future.

As for next steps, we will continue to work with DOD and the Presidential Advisory Committee to help get answers to these important questions. We are also prepared to address your questions after this briefing.

Now, let's do a little bit of history. Let me summarize our findings briefly. First, we continue to believe, on the basis of a comprehensive review of intelligence, that Iraq did not deploy chemical or biological weapons in Kuwait or use them during the Gulf War. Second, analysis and computer modeling indicate chemical agents released by aerial bombing of chemical warfare facilities in northern Iraq did not reach U.S. troops in Saudi Arabia. Finally, our review surfaced evidence that CW agents had been released at two separate locations near Khamisiyah in southern Iraq as a result of demolition activity.

What is new since our last appearance before you is that we have worked with an expert group to evaluate the methodologies used in modeling efforts. This is the group requested by then DCI Deutch and convened by Deputy Secretary of Defense John White. To this end, DOD has asked the Institute of Defense Analysis to convene a panel drawn from the scientific and technical community. The panel first met in late November and we anticipate its final report shortly for release to the public.

Let me take a moment, Mr. Chairman, to review CIA's role in analyzing Iraq's chemical and biological weapons programs to help put into context our participation in investigating U.S. exposure to chemical weapons. I will break my remarks in three parts: Our intelligence focus before, during, and after the war.

The Intelligence Community has long followed Iraq's chemical and biological programs as part of its mission to assess chemical and biological weapons capabilities worldwide. Before the war, CIA, like others in the Intelligence Community, assessed that Iraq had a significant chemical and biological weapons capability, including chemically armed SCUDS. We also assessed that Iraq had used chemical weapons on numerous occasions against Iran and its own citizens. The Intelligence Community at the time had reached a consensus that Iraq had chemical weapons in its arsenal, had forward deployed these weapons, and was prepared to use them against coalition forces.

During the war as Desert Storm began, our concerns about Iraqi use of weapons of mass destruction became the foremost focus of our chemical and biological weapons analytic and collection efforts. Our analysts, in cooperation with their colleagues in other agencies, sought to identify possible Iraqi CW and BW facilities for targeting purposes. In all, 32 sites were identified, albeit based on incomplete and sometimes inaccurate information. And it is important to note that at this point in time we did not identify Khamisiyah as such a site. A key objective for both military and intelligence personnel was the early detection of the use of chemical and biological weapons. We received several reports of detection alarms. CIA operated a 24-hour chemical and biological detection unit at the start of the air war and maintained it through the ground campaign to monitor and assess such reports.

In the months immediately after the war, we turned our intelligence assets to identifying and characterizing Iraq's CW and BW capabilities. The primary focus of our efforts during 1993 and 1994 consisted of supporting UNSCOM inspections, assessing Iraq's declarations of issues of weapons of mass destruction, refining collection requirements, and interpreting intelligence to attempt to root out remaining Iraqi CW capabilities. During this time, CIA also worked with DOD to try to track down and check the validity of possible causes of chemical detections that occurred during the war. A good example of this was the 19 January 1991 Czech detection of nerve agents in Saudi Arabia. In this case, we sent an analyst to Czechoslovakia to further research the claim. We also had our contractor modeler look at the possible causes for detection. We concluded that the detections were credible due to the specificity of the equipment and the quality of the procedures used by the Czechs. However, we were unable to conclusively determine the cause. We nonetheless remain convinced that the presence of chemical agents was not due to Iraqi offensive actions such as the use of SCUD missiles.

In March of 1995, CIA began a thorough reexamination of the relevant intelligence. We did so because of the President's concern and because of questions that were raised by CIA employees. This review culminated in the publication of our report last August. Let me address head on a question that is probably on your mind, one that's been asked today—why didn't CIA and the Intelligence Community focus on potential exposure earlier. A number of reasons contributed to the gap between 1991 and March of 1995 when we began the intelligence review. From the beginning, the consensus within the U.S. Government was that Iraq had not used chemical or biological weapons during the war. Analysis since then has maintained that view. Moreover, Iraq engaged in widespread deception with regard to where it stored its chemical weapons; therefore, many reports received during this time were viewed with great skepticism by our analysts. UNSCOM could not in 1991 corroborate that a demolition had occurred at the facility at Khamisiyah.

Shortly after the war, the conditions now commonly referred to as Gulf War illness had not been widely reported to us. As a result, our intelligence requirements did not make it a priority at the time to examine all incidence of potential low level exposure. In these circumstances, we focused on support to UNSCOM. When we did focus more broadly on potential exposures short of Iraqi use, we identified two primary scenarios—fallout from the aerial bombings in Iraq, or fallout from demolition activity in the Kuwaiti theater of operations.

Let me turn first to the fallout from the aerial bombings. Based on currently available information, we conclude that Coalition air bombing damaged filled chemical munitions at two facilities, Muhammadiyat and Al Muthanna. Both are located in remote areas of west Baghdad. At the request of the Presidential Advisory Committee, CIA had modeled releases from these facilities. That modeling indicates that fallout from these facilities did not reach our troops in Saudi Arabia.

Turning to the potential exposure in the Kuwaiti Theater of Operations, we now know that on 4 March 1991 U.S. troops destroyed nerve agent filled with 122mm rockets in Bunker 73 at Khamisiyah. On 10 March 1991, they also destroyed CW rockets at the pit area near Khamisiyah. UNSCOM inspected chemical munitions at or near Khamisiyah in October of 1991. The Iraqis claimed during the October 1991 inspection that coalition troops had destroyed the bunker earlier that year. We viewed the Iraqi statements with skepticism at the time because of Baghdad's widespread use of deception against UNSCOM, because we then had so little other intelligence to confirm the Iraqi assertion, and because UNSCOM itself could not verify that chemical weapons had been destroyed until 1996.

We came back to Khamisiyah though, even with all of these doubts, in 1995. We narrowed in on this as a place that we had to return for further analysis. We asked for DOD's investigative team to look into whether troops were there. We researched the issue together and by early 1996 CIA and DOD had developed information that enabled us to believe that U.S. troops did, in fact, blow up Bunker 73. The potential exposure of U.S. troops was confirmed on 10 March. On that day a CIA analyst heard a tape recording of a radio show in which a veteran of the 37th Engineering Battalion described demolition activities at a facility that the analyst immediately recognized as Khamisiyah. On May 1 we briefed the Presidential Advisory Committee.

Any remaining doubts that the weapons were chemical were removed by an UNSCOM inspection in May of 1996. The UNSCOM inspectors documented the presence of high density polyethylene inserts and other material that proved this point. In addition, during the inspection the Iraqis gave us a great deal of other information that for the first time we were able to independently corroborate from other sources of information. We published this information as well as the results of the modeling of the down-wind hazard. These results, as well as the results of the modeling at Muhammadiyat and Al Muthanna are available on the Internet.

Mr. Chairman, I'll stop there. However, if you were to ask me what was the lesson learned here, we did a good job before the war of understanding the Iraqi threat, and we did a very good job of providing intelligence to folks during the conduct of this war. After the war, we all—the entire Defense and Intelligence Communities—could have done a much better job of focusing and integrating information on both sides of the house that would have lead us to an earlier understanding of many of these events. We didn't get there soon enough. When we got there in 1995, we—this Agency and the Intelligence Community—aggressively pursued every bit of information we could. We have released as much of it as we can to the public, and we intend to continue to do so. Thank you.

[The prepared statement of Mr. Tenet appears on page 78.]

Chairman SPECTER. Thank you very much, Director Tenet. The key issue is how to take care of the veterans who were exposed to whatever problems there were in the Gulf War. And the secondary issue, as I outlined at the start, is what has been the response of the Department of Defense and other executive agencies. We are concerned as to what DOD did. Was it indifference? Was it carelessness? Was it recklessness? Was it a cover-up? That we intend to pursue in depth.

Senator Rockefeller has used the expression "reckless disregard." I just told him that there are legal doctrines which classify reckless disregard and elevate it to a form of intentional wrongdoing. For example, reckless disregard of the safety of another person can rise to murder in the second degree. Reckless disregard in a liable context can be equated under Sullivan v. New York Times with malice, with what is intentional wrongdoing. We are going to ascertain as best we can just what the Department of Defense did, whether it was intentional, whether it was reckless, or whether it was a cover-up.

The United Nations teams, according to information provided to us, had information about the potential exposure of chemical warfare from Khamisiyah way back in 1991 on this occurrence from March of 1991. When was it that it first came to the attention in a digestible form by CIA?

Mr. TENET. When did we first issue the report?

Ms. COPELAND. The inspection occurred in October 1991. We got the report sometime in November. It was issued throughout the U.S. Government. We viewed that report with skepticism as did the inspectors. They reported what they were told by the Iraqis but even they did not believe it. They thought that they had been deceived by the Iraqis.

Chairman SPECTER. So the CIA knew in October of 1991 that there had been a destruction of chemical components in March of 1991?

Ms. COPELAND. What we were told was that there were chemical munitions found at Khamisiyah. The Iraqis also told UNSCOM inspectors that there had been demolition activity by coalition forces at a bunker called 73. That's the information we had. The UNSCOM inspectors were not able to corroborate that information and were skeptical of it, and we were skeptical of it and were not able to corroborate it.

Chairman SPECTER. Well, you had the information, you were skeptical of it, you could not corroborate it, but you could not disprove it either.

Ms. COPELAND. That's correct.

Mr. TENET. And we disseminated the information.

Chairman SPECTER. And you disseminated the information to the Department of Defense in October of 1991?

Mr. TENET. We disseminated it throughout the United States Government at the time.

Ms. COPELAND. November.

Chairman SPECTER. Well, the Department of Defense is a part of the United States Government.

Mr. TENET. The last time I looked, yes.

Chairman SPECTER. Okay. Then skipping ahead, what happened immediately preceding June of 1996 when the Department of Defense finally made the dissemination? Do you know what caused the Department of Defense finally to own up that there had been chemical detonation at Khamisiyah in June of 1996?

Mr. TENET. Senator, I can't speak to what made them own up to it. I can only tell you that we had undertaken beginning in March of 1995 a comprehensive assessment of—

Chairman SPECTER. All right. My preceding question was what occurred prior to June of 1996 which might account for their disclosure, and then I asked the simplistic question and you gave me an accurate answer that you can't look inside the minds of DOD. Okay. But in trying to retrace the steps, something occurred which called it to their attention in a forceful way immediately prior to their finally owning up that there had been this detonation. What was that?

Ms. SLATKIN. As the Acting Director was starting to say, Mr. Chairman, we began a comprehensive review in March of 1995. In September of 1995, as we were comprehensively reviewing all of our intelligence, our analysts got enough information to identify three different sites. At that time they identified Khamisiyah as one of the more interesting sites to continue to look at because of its proximity to coalition forces. We continued to investigate that event, events surrounding Khamisiyah.

Chairman SPECTER. Did the Department of Defense know you were undertaking that intense investigation at that time?

Ms. SLATKIN. Everyone in the United States Government began to reevaluate all their information in March of 1995.

Chairman SPECTER. Ms. Slatkin, with all due respect, that kind of a statement doesn't help us very much. Everyone in the United States Government began to reevaluate, that doesn't say much. Not everyone in the United States Government did that.

Ms. SLATKIN. Mr. Chairman, as you recall in March of 1995, President Clinton initiated a major review inside the Department of Defense. Our review was also initiated at that time.

Chairman SPECTER. Okay. So Defense was involved in it, CIA was involved in it. What I'm looking at specifically is what Defense was doing at that time.

Ms. SLATKIN. Sir, I can't speak for what the Department of Defense was doing at that time. But I would like to tell you how we learned about the Khamisiyah event.

Chairman SPECTER. Please proceed.

Ms. SLATKIN. And then when and how we provided that information, because I believe that is what you're trying to get at.

Chairman SPECTER. Go ahead.

Ms. SLATKIN. On March 10, as Mr. Tenet has said, we identified Khamisiyah as one of the sites we ought to pay attention to. On March 10, one of our CIA analysts, Larry Fox, who is one of our chemical weapons analysts, is working on this problem, hears the tape of a veteran from the 37th Engineer Battalion talking about a demolition at a site in Iraq. It becomes clear to him that that is the same facility that he's been looking at inside the CIA as one of the three sites, Khamisiyah.

As soon as we learned that information, we immediately in March go to the Department of Defense and notify them that we have put together pieces of the puzzle that Khamisiyah is a site, and Khamisiyah is a site where we ought to go back and say who was there, what activity was underway. That happens in March. The next day we go to the Department of Defense and we notify them of that information.

Chairman SPECTER. Precisely whom did you notify at the Department of Defense?

Ms. SLATKIN. We went to the Persian Gulf investigative team, to the head of the Persian Gulf investigative team.

Chairman SPECTER. And the identity of that person is?

Ms. SLATKIN. They report to Dr. Steve Joseph in the Department of Defense.

Ms. COPELAND. Right, but they talked to the Persian Gulf investigative team.

Senator ROCKEFELLER. Not anymore they don't. [Laughter.]

Ms. COPELAND. They did at that time, Senator. We told one of the lieutenant colonels who was one of the investigators. So it was our analyst talking to another one of their investigators. We talk to them regularly. Whenever we find anything we let them know, and they let us know of findings. So it was as part of our continuing exchange, and it immediately happened the next day after the analyst heard this taped show.

Ms. SLATKIN. On May 1, Sylvia Copeland testified before the Presidential Advisory Committee that Dr. Lashof heads, and she announced during that testimony publicly that we had credible evidence that U.S. troops unwittingly destroyed chemical weapons. On May 22, as Mr. Tenet pointed out, UNSCOM inspected Khamisiyah. That allowed us to document for the first time the presence of munitions. It allowed us to put that together with all the other information. And that is when it was abundantly clear what had happened at Khamisiyah.

In early June, we again briefed the Department of Defense, the Persian Gulf investigative team, as well as the Presidential Advisory Committee. On June 21 those results were announced publicly by the Department of Defense, as you well know.

Chairman SPECTER. Okay. That's a chronology which we'll be taking a very close look at.

Senator Rockefeller?

Senator ROCKEFELLER. Thank you, Mr. Chairman. I'm going to make a little statement, and then any of you who want to respond to this, fine. Mr. Tenet, as you know, I have a very high regard for you. This is a different subject somewhat. You know of my frustration. When CIA says we don't know the mind of DOD, I don't believe that. When DOD says we don't know the mind of CIA, I don't believe that.

In other words, everybody is off in their separate pockets protecting themselves, and I reject that type of thinking.

It will come as no surprise to you that I am, at the very least, appalled by the inability of the Department of Defense to recover some mysteriously missing pages of the NBC, which is the nuclear/biological/chemical logs that were maintained during the war. There is a gap in there of 8 days which somehow disappeared. Usually when one loses logs one loses all of logs, but in this case only 8 days of logs were lost, including the time of Khamisiyah and perhaps one of the other explosions. The effect of this—whether it is fact or illusion—is that DOD appears to have been withholding important information from the American public, and the CIA appears to have failed to recognize, to get inside the mind of DOD—failed to underscore, failed to communicate. I don't know how to explain it, but I know critical information was lost at a time that it was, and is, needed.

This is extremely important information for this Committee and the American people to provide for a full accounting of what happened at Khamisiyah. But, Director Tenet, were you aware that there was another totally separate record that was being kept of these events by General Schwarzkopf—the so-called XO or Executive Officer logs?

Mr. TENET. No, sir.

Senator ROCKEFELLER. You were not aware?

Mr. TENET. No, sir, I'm not aware.

Sylvia, were you aware?

Ms. COPELAND. No.

Senator ROCKEFELLER. I am further appalled. These were totally different from the NBC logs. An Executive Officer followed General Schwarzkopf around everywhere he went, taking down every single possible thing that happened during every single moment of his very, very long and stressful days. The Schwarzkopf XO logs contain very detailed notes which were taken continuously, as I indicated, by an Executive Officer assigned to him for the express purpose of providing the general with a record of every meeting, every briefing, every conversation in the Gulf that was in any way related to the war. The inspector general of the Department of Defense says that these logs that I now refer to were intended to serve as the General's personal record to refresh his memory regarding his decisions and conversations. And in at least nine instances, again, the inspector general avowed that the General intended the log to be exclusively for his own personal use.

Now, I am not so suspicious as to ever think that these logs would have been held separately for the possibility of writing a book. [Laughter.] But I will tell you that the acting archivist of the United States of America, Trudy Peterson, said that these logs fit the definition of Federal records as defined in the Records Disposal Act. In other words, this is a very serious matter and a very serious log which is at the General's disposal and evidently not your's or the DOD's.

My first question was were you aware of the logs, and your answer was no. Has the CIA, or will the CIA ask General Schwarzkopf to provide these logs as part of your investigation now that you do know?

Mr. TENET. At this point, Senator, what we're doing is supporting inquiries that the DOD is pursuing with regards to—

Senator ROCKEFELLER. Why don't you just say yes, George, that you'll put in a request for them. I wrote Deputy Secretary John D. White about these XO logs on December 6, Mr. Chairman, and I was extremely honored to get back a letter of two paragraphs from somebody named Kimberly Clausen who deals with pols like myself, because she's called a "Congressional Actions Coordinator," saying that an inquiry into this matter has been initiated.

[Senator Rockefeller's 12/6/96 letter to Deputy Secretary White appears on page 115.]

Chairman SPECTER. Senator Rockefeller, don't pay any attention to the time. Go ahead.

Mr. TENET. Senator, if there is information in those logs that bear on what we're trying to do, we will of course try to access that information.

Senator ROCKEFELLER. I cannot believe that you didn't know about it. I cannot believe it. And Ms. Slatkin, I've watched you on television and you can handle any question and turn everything in the right direction. How could you not know about this separate log?

Ms. SLATKIN. Senator, this is the first I've heard that General Schwarzkopf kept a separate log.

Senator ROCKEFELLER. Of every single thing that happened every single day. Which means that the probability—now, I happen to think that those 8 days were disposed of for ill purposes. That's my prejudice. I don't know that. I have no proof of that. That's my view. But certainly those 8 days are going to be covered by the XO log. What are you going to do with this information?

Ms. SLATKIN. As you know, Senator, those missing 8 days are critical to our understanding of the modeling effort we've been asked to undertake at the pit area. Our problem in modeling the pit area was the fact that we had so much uncertainty. We were uncertain about the dates—

Senator ROCKEFELLER. Well, here's a lot less uncertainty which is potentially available to you.

Ms. SLATKIN. Yes, sir.

Mr. TENET. We'll pursue it, Senator.

Senator ROCKEFELLER. You're going to pursue it?

Mr. TENET. Yes, sir.

Senator ROCKEFELLER. You're going to try to get it. Obviously, you didn't have access to these logs during your investigation since you didn't know about them.

Mr. Chairman, I thank you.

Chairman SPECTER. Thank you very much, Senator Rockefeller. Senator Jeffords?

Senator JEFFORDS. Mr. Chairman, I have no questions for this panel. I'll be waiting for the next panel.

Chairman SPECTER. Thank you very much, Director Tenet, Ms. Slatkin, and Ms. Copeland.

Mr. TENET. Thank you, sir.

Chairman SPECTER. The logs which Senator Rockefeller has referred to are of obvious importance. We will await further developments as you pursue them. We appreciate your being here.

Mr. TENET. Thank you.

Chairman SPECTER. I would like to now call the next panel of Dr. Joyce Lashof and her assistants. Dr. Joyce C. Lashof is the distinguished Chairperson of the Presidential Advisory Committee on Gulf War Veterans' Illnesses. She is the former dean and professor emeritus of the School of Public Health at the University of California at Berkeley. She had a distinguished record in public service as assistant director of the Office of Technology Assessment in 1978 through 1981, had been the Deputy Assistant Secretary for Health Programs, and Deputy Assistant Secretary for Population Affairs previous to that at the Department of Health, Education, and Welfare. She served from 1991 to 1992 as president of the American Public Health Association.

Senator Rockefeller and I had the pleasure of hearing her report to the President day before yesterday. She is joined today by a member of the board, Dr. Philip J. Landrigan, who is the Ethel H. Wise professor and chairman of the Department of Community Medicine at Mount Sinai Medical Center in New York. Welcome to you as well, Dr. Landrigan.

Mr. LANDRIGAN. Thank you, Mr. Chairman.

Ms. LASHOF. Dr. Landrigan is a member of our presidential advisory committee and I've asked him to assist me today.

Chairman SPECTER. Very good. We appreciate your making time from your busy schedule to be with us today, Dr. Lashof. The floor is yours. To the extent you can summarize within the 10-minute time limit, we would appreciate it.

STATEMENT OF JOYCE C. LASHOF, M.D., CHAIRPERSON, THE PRESIDENTIAL ADVISORY COMMITTEE ON

PERSIAN GULF WAR VETERANS' ILLNESSES ACCOMPANIED BY PHILIP J. LANDRIGAN, M.D., MEMBER, PRESIDENTIAL ADVISORY COMMITTEE ON PERSIAN GULF WAR VETERANS' ILLNESSES, CHAIRMAN, DEPARTMENT OF COMMUNITY MEDICINE, MOUNT SINAI MEDICAL CENTER, NEW YORK

Dr. LASHOF. Thank you very much, Mr. Chairman, and members of the Committee, Senator Rockefeller. I appreciate the opportunity to be here today. As you know, our final report was released to the President earlier this week. We have submitted the report's executive summary as our written testimony for the record, and we of course have supplied you with the copy of the full report. As you requested, Dr. Landrigan and I will now summarize that material.

Before turning things over to Dr. Landrigan, who will discuss the committee's work specifically in the area of health effects, risk factors, research and investigation, I would like to make a few general observations. First, there should be no question that the committee recognizes that many veterans are experiencing medical problems connected to their service in the Gulf. In the near term, the Government needs to fine tune some specific efforts in followup clinical care and in risk communication. Overall, however, the committee believed that the Government had learned some lessons from our experience in Vietnam and we were encouraged for the most part by the Government's response to the range of health related problems experienced by Gulf veterans.

With that, I will turn it over to Dr. Landrigan to discuss some specific areas and then I will make some final comments about what we think needs to be done in the future to prevent this kind of thing again.

Chairman SPECTER. Thank you very much for those comments, Dr. Lashof. We now turn to Dr. Landrigan.

Dr. LANDRIGAN. Thank you, Mr. Chairman. There is no question, sir, that many thousands of the 697,000 men and women who went to the Gulf have come back ill. Some of them have specific illnesses such as leishmaniasis and malaria that clearly relate to their service and are relatively straightforward to diagnose. But there are many thousands more people who were exposed to a range of toxic exposures as well as psychological and physiologic stress who have returned home with a whole raft of symptoms and illnesses that you've enumerated this morning. Many of these symptoms and illnesses defy ready diagnostic classification despite a very extensive portfolio of research.

I think at this point our committee feels comfortable in drawing a series of conclusions about illness in Gulf War veterans. The first is the most obvious, and that is that there is no question whatsoever that these people are suffering, that their illness is real, that they've been made sick. We're gratified that there is not an increased number of deaths in these veterans. We're gratified that there have not been an increased number hospitalized. Nevertheless, it remains indubitable that there is more illness in them than expected.

The second point is that somewhat to our chagrin we have to acknowledge that current scientific evidence simply does not support a causal link between any of the particular exposures that the veterans experienced and the illness that they are experiencing. We reviewed a whole series of potential exposures which included extremes of heat and cold, blowing dust, smoke from the oil well fires, petroleum fuels, pyridostigmine bromide, the vaccines, depleted uranium, chemical warfare agents, pesticides. We would like to be able to pin disease on some of those factors, but a combination of inadequate baseline data on the veterans before they went out, inadequate measures of exposures that were incurred during and after the war, and in some cases lack of research results simply make it impossible to prove cause and effect relationships. I was at the JAMA press conference yesterday because I was the author of an editorial that was in the same issue of JAMA as the Haley and the CDC papers. What I said then I will repeat today. I think that the papers from Texas raise some interesting questions, those were elegant and sophisticated studies, but in my view they don't prove the point. They raise the question, they suggest the urgent need for some further research which is what the Committee calls for.

Finally, I think we all have to acknowledge that stress is a very important factor here. None of us are saying that stress is the only factor, but stress is important. Extreme stress that was experienced by the veterans over a period of the many months that they were in the Gulf area can play out in the succeeding years in a number of ways. It can play out as heart disease, as hypertension, as psychological and psychiatric disease, as multiple chemical sensitivity. It can make itself manifest in many ways. We were at great pains to emphasize the notion that runs through all of medicine, that mind and body are not separated, that damage that is done to the mind can play out in damage to the body, and indeed vice versa.

We also identified important data gaps and we made specific recommendations for further research. One area of research that clearly needs to be pursued and pursued aggressively is the whole issue of what are the chronic effects of relatively low level exposure to chemical warfare agents. The Committee recommend more research in that area. Some research is now underway at the VA centers in Portland, Oregon, Boston, and some work is going on in Japan among survivors of the subway attacks. But that research portfolio needs to be expanded. I understand that with the new money that the DoD and

VA are going to put on the street it will be. We also think that the large population-based studies such as the Iowa study and the VA National Health Survey will yield additional information. Clearly, those studies need to be pursued aggressively.

Overall, our committee was reasonably well satisfied with the portfolio of research that DOD and the VA have underway and are contemplating. But as we have said and has been widely noted, our committee took strong issue with the Government's performance in one key area and we were very much disappointed by the DOD's failure to act in good faith on the whole issue of the investigation of possible exposure of the troops to chemical and biological weapons.

Chairman SPECTER. What you just said there is very important, Dr. Landrigan. Let me interrupt you if I may. Your conclusion that the Department of Defense did not operate in good faith, would you amplify why you concluded that the Department of Defense did not operate in good faith.

Dr. LANDRIGAN. Yes, sir. It is our feeling that the information was not aggressively pursued and it was not made known early enough to enable health researchers to focus earlier on on the question of chronic health effects that might have been due to those agents.

Chairman SPECTER. Specifically, what information did the Department of Defense not pass on to health experts?

Dr. LANDRIGAN. Let me answer it this way, that our committee is very, very proud of the fact that investigators from our committee were the people who pushed and pushed and pushed on the DOD to make the DOD go back and examine their records and finally come forward with the information that the exposures to the chemical warfare agents had occurred at Khamisiyah.

Chairman SPECTER. Absent that push and push and push from the presidential committee, the Department of Defense would not have come forward with that evidence?

Dr. LANDRIGAN. May not have, or may not have come forward even when they did, yes, sir.

Chairman SPECTER. Well, they certainly hadn't on their own.

Dr. LANDRIGAN. That is correct.

Chairman SPECTER. And when you pressed them they finally did.

Dr. LANDRIGAN. Yes, sir.

Chairman SPECTER. Precisely what did the committee do to press Department of Defense on that matter?

Dr. LASHOF. If I may.

Chairman SPECTER. Madam Chairman?

Dr. LASHOF. Thank you. Members of our staff investigated matters, looking at the whole issue of chemical and biological weapons. One member learned very early from CIA that there were 3 areas that they were looking at and Khamisiyah was one of them. He pursued that, asked for more information, was briefed regularly by CIA—

Chairman SPECTER. Who was that individual, Dr. Lashof?

Dr. LASHOF. Jim Turner. He asked CIA to testify, as Ms. Slatkin indicated a little while ago, at the May meeting of our committee following a subcommittee meeting in Atlanta in April to look specifically at the issue of chemical and biological weapons. CIA presented information at both meetings. We then had a full meeting of the full committee in July and we requested that DoD and CIA present at the July meeting their knowledge and understanding of what happened at Khamisiyah. DoD had a press conference just before our meeting to release that information since they knew they would be releasing it to our committee. We certainly felt that we precipitated the release at that time. I don't think we can really comment on when they would have released it if we had not pushed them.

Chairman SPECTER. Well, it is sufficient that you precipitated it.

Dr. LASHOF. I think that is correct.

Chairman SPECTER. At least that causal connection has been established. Now we have to go on to the causal connection between chemical exposure and the problems faced by the Gulf War veterans. I interrupted you. Please proceed, Dr. Landrigan.

Dr. LANDRIGAN. That really concluded my portion, Mr. Chairman. I think Dr. Lashof had a few concluding words.

Chairman SPECTER. Please proceed, Dr. Lashof.

Dr. LASHOF. Thank you. On the last point you just raised, I'm not sure Dr. Landrigan made clear that as a result of that we did say that one of our recommendations is further research on the effects of low level chemical exposure and that the data on that are not adequate.

Some general other things I'd like to mention, however. During the course of our analyses specific to Gulf War veterans' illness, it became apparent that the Government could do a better job in the future preventing post-conflict concerns generally. Therefore, the committee also recommended that a Presidential Review Directive be issued to instruct the National Science and Technology Council to develop an interagency plan to address health preparedness for and readjustment of veterans and families after future conflicts and peacekeeping missions. This plan would need to have extensive external review and it should address the need for better communication, better data, and better services.

I would like to highlight a few of the specific recommendations we made in the area of communication and data. First, the Government clearly needs to work on better communication with our servicemen and women. The committee recommends that DoD and VA develop and implement a comprehensive risk communication plan and that they solicit timely and public expert testimony and comment on any rule that permits waiver of informed consent for use of investigational products in military exigencies.

The Government needs better data. Many of the health concerns of Gulf War veterans may never be resolved fully because of the lack of data. To help prevent similar problems in the future, we recommend that a high priority be assigned to dealing with the problem of lost or missing records. The Government needs to develop a protocol for a thorough health evaluation on a large sample of troops to enable better post-deployment medical epidemiology. We believe research on possible causes and methods of prevention of excess mortality from external causes among veterans deserves attention as well.

Finally, we recommend obtaining data via routine surveys of the reproductive health of military populations.

In the area of better services, the committee recommended that the Government seek statutory authority to treat veterans and their families for service connective reproductive problems. And because society at large continues to stigmatize mental health concerns, we recommend that the Government continue and intensify efforts to develop stress reduction programs for all troops with special emphasis on deployed troops.

In conclusion, Mr. Chairman, Senator Rockefeller, Senator Jeffords, in many important ways the Nation has begun to pay its debt to Gulf veterans. It is essential now that we move swiftly towards resolving the principal remaining concerns—how many troops were exposed to chemical warfare agents and to what degree, and did that exposure indeed contribute to illness.

I thank you for the opportunity to review our work with you. We're prepared to answer your questions, I hope.

[The referenced executive summary appear on pages 85.]

Chairman SPECTER. Thank you very much, Dr. Lashof. You and your committee have done an outstanding job and we appreciate the service you've rendered and your willingness to go forward as the President has made that request to you.

My question to you, Dr. Landrigan, picks up on your testimony that the studies yesterday did not prove the point. I had a chance to talk to Dr. Haley very briefly. As he went through a number of what he characterized as syndromes, it is my understanding, we're going to have to have him testify and go through the whole process, and we intend to do that, that he found what he classified as syndrome II where Gulf War veterans couldn't work, they lost their balance, the room was spinning, that they had taken the PB tablets, the anti-nerve tablets, and the bromide and, if taken after the fact, there were side effects. At least as I understood, he felt that the people in syndrome II were causally related to exposure to chemical warfare.

I note in the report you conclude that "the evidence of chemical warfare agent release at Khamisiyah is overwhelming and low level exposure to troops within a 50 kilometer radius should be presumed." What does it take, Dr. Landrigan, in your medical judgment to establish the causal connection, the proof of the point so to speak?

Dr. LANDRIGAN. Let me begin by saying I have a lot of respect for Dr. Haley. He and I actually served together for 5 or 6 years at the Centers for Disease Control. We were both in the Public Health Service together down there. He's a good researcher.

I have no question about his findings in regard to the symptoms in these men. He evaluated them very carefully and got good, accurate information. I believe he is on somewhat thinner ground when he gets into the details of cause and effect and there's a couple of reasons. The first is that exposures were self-reported. The second is that only 41 percent of the Seabee battalion whom he was examining participated. It was a low participation rate as these surveys go. And then it was only an even smaller fraction, 23 men in total, who came forward for the detailed neurophysiologic exams that they did down in Texas. But having said that, none of that is to take away from the quality of what they did. My feeling is that what they need to do now before they can generalize findings on 23 veterans to a larger population is that they've got to do detailed studies on a larger population.

Chairman SPECTER. But as to the 23, was the conclusion sound?

Dr. LANDRIGAN. It's sound as far as it goes, sir. But it is awfully hard to generalize to a group of 700,000 people from the experience of 23. You just need a bigger sample than that. Even people that are used to Nielsen polls with 1 or 2 percent of a population sample would agree I think that 23 is not enough to generalize to the whole group. That's the fundamental problem.

Chairman SPECTER. How big a group do you need?

Dr. LANDRIGAN. I can't answer off the top of my head, but there are established procedures for getting there. You basically take a valid sample of those who participated and include in that sample sufficient statistical power to get valid results. There are well-known ways that statisticians get there.

Chairman SPECTER. But would you accept the conclusion as to those 23, that there was cause and effect?

Dr. LANDRIGAN. I would accept that Dr. Haley has done a very good job of putting the question at center stage. I don't think he has sufficiently answered the question.

Chairman SPECTER. But how about as to those 23? If you're saying that the sample ought to be bigger, I don't think the logic holds as to a bigger sampling as, for example, on a public opinion poll. But putting that aside, if you have the 23 and Dr. Haley's work was sound, was his conclusion as to cause and effect accurate as to those 23 whom he did examine?

Dr. LANDRIGAN. I think the really central problem here is one of selectivity. Only 40 percent participated in the first place, and only a tiny subset of them came to the final study. So it is hard to know who these people are, what they represent. It's just a fundamental precept in epidemiologic studies that you have to work with a representative population. These people, by definition, are not representative. They can't be, not given the way they were chosen.

Chairman SPECTER. All right. Let's accept your conclusion that they're not representative. But as to themselves, does the conclusion of cause and effect apply as to those 23 individuals?

Dr. LANDRIGAN. Unfortunately, the study is just not really set up to answer it with regard to 23 people.

Dr. LASHOF. Let me try also to get into this.

Chairman SPECTER. Dr. Lashof.

Dr. LASHOF. Phil did review it and wrote the editorial. I looked at the study relatively briefly last night so I don't want to talk about the quality of the work from that point of view, but rather try to explain what it is Dr. Landrigan is saying about 23 people from this. There are no specific data as to the exposure of these 23. It's self-reported. The subjects believe they were in an area where risk factors were, but nothing was measured, so there is no real exposure data. And as I understand it, the basis of making the conclusion that it is related to this was a statistical basis, saying that X number of people who responded to the survey said such and such happened and from that group we drew some conclusions based on more having said they were exposed who had this particular finding. But if the sample isn't right, you can't validly generalize. Haley doesn't have a cause and effect in that he has specific data that these 23 people said they had this exposure and this exposure causes this kind of illness, as we might if you had a pneumococcus floating around in your blood. There wasn't a specific thing he could identify in these individuals. So he was making the judgment based on statistical conclusions drawn from his larger sample. I don't know if that muddies the water for you, but I think that's what Dr. Landrigan was trying to get at when he was getting into a description of epidemiologic techniques and statistics.

Chairman SPECTER. Is that what you were trying to get at, Dr. Landrigan?

Dr. LANDRIGAN. Yes, sir. Maybe a good way to amplify this and say the same thing is through analogy. A lot of my life has been spent doing studies of occupational disease—asbestos, lead poisoning, benzene, and the like. The most difficult part of those studies is to document the exposure. In the populations exposed to benzene, for example, it's been easy to diagnose leukemia and lymphoma in the survivors of exposure, but it took us almost a decade to properly quantify exposure and develop solid dose response relationships that were accepted by the courts. The assessment of exposure is always the most difficult thing in these retrospective studies, particularly in a case like this where the chemical sarin leaves no chemical footprint in the human body. You can't take a blood sample and find a trace of sarin. It's gone. It's evanescent.

Chairman SPECTER. Well, I'll let Senator Rockefeller pursue this line, if he chooses to.

Senator ROCKEFELLER. I'd be happy to, Mr. Chairman. I regret the concentration on the number 23. I started working on this thing 4 years ago and we put out a report which is good, I think. The Department of Defense, when they decided to use pyridostigmine bromide, did two studies—one involved 28 people, the other involved 32. On the basis of that, they went ahead and ordered pyridostigmine for the whole population. In one of those cases, one of the people who took PB passed out on the spot; in the other case I'm not sure what happened, but it was something bad. But they went ahead and did it. So I don't want to get hung up on numbers.

I understand, Doctor, you said that the Texas research was ambitious and sophisticated. You also said it raises the possibility of toxic exposure as a cause of the disease, but that in your opinion it does not pin it to the ground. I totally agree. So what we're really saying is that we don't know so far what this multiplicity of interactions might be. But that's all we're saying so far. And Dr. Lashof said we've got to do much more research, we're just beginning; I think the President said we're at the beginning of the road. Believe me, we're at the beginning of the road. But we've got to get down it so we can help these people and prevent this from ever happening again in future wars which are going to be like this.

As I mentioned in my opening statement, the concentration—and I did you some disservice, Dr. Lashof, because you didn't just say stress, there were other things that you talked about—but I was troubled by the focus on stress. I felt that there was a focus on stress at the expense of perhaps other things, for example, the combination of what happens when you mix insecticides like DEET with pyridostigmine bromide. And this doesn't fit my point, but it is an absolutely stunning fact, Mr. Chairman, that the Department of Defense chose to give pyridostigmine bromide as a sort of pretreatment which in itself is an investigational drug not approved by the FDA, for which they got a waiver, and which has no effect unless it's also given with atropine and

2-PAM, which they didn't do. And if they had done it, it would have been effective against soman, which we know that the Iraqis did not have. They had sarin. This is the most incredible stupidity of trying to prepare our troops against chemical exposures that I can ever dream of—something which they wrongly gave for a chemical weapon which the Iraqis did not have and we knew it.

Leaving that aside, I get back to this question of stress and this overriding focus on psychological conditions. A couple of questions about this. The clinical evaluations of DOD—the CCEP study—found, as has been mentioned, 36 percent of Gulf War veterans evaluated had "psychological conditions." But isn't it also true that 47 percent of the veterans exhibited symptoms of musculoskeletal system disease, and 43 percent were found to have what DOD calls "symptoms, signs, and ill-defined conditions," a classification which sounds to me like undiagnosed illnesses? Is that correct?

Dr. LASHOF. Yes, that is correct. That is exactly what that term is used for.

Senator ROCKEFELLER. Isn't it also true that the category of "psychological conditions," while containing some valid diagnoses such as depression, also included more clearly defined physical symptoms such as tension headaches?

Dr. LASHOF. Yes.

Senator ROCKEFELLER. Given the significant level, which bothers me as I've indicated, of the interpretation of clinical findings and the strong focus on psychological conditions in the explanation of Gulf War illnesses, is there a mental health specialist such as a clinical psychologist or psychiatrist on the presidential advisory committee?

Dr. LASHOF. Absolutely. Dr. David Hamburg, one of the most preeminent psychiatrists in this country.

Senator ROCKEFELLER. Was he a staff member or a member?

Dr. LASHOF. A member of the committee.

Senator ROCKEFELLER. He's very good. OK. I think one of the great tragedies of all this, Mr. Chairman, is that we have been distracted so much by the Khamisiyah events. That has been a wonderful excuse for people to get away from, in my opinion at least, the original problems that we're talking about, which was pyridostigmine bromide, the research of Dr. Moss which showed that if you mixed that with insecticides, i.e., DEET, which certainly was happening out there, it increased the effect of PB by as much 10 times. He was fired from the U.S. Department of Agriculture for conducting such research and is still unemployed somewhere. And Dr. Abou-Donia's research tended to back up this type of thing.

In other words, it's interesting to me that the research that DOD has done and that the VA has done has failed to establish—and in some sense you all backed or agreed with this—failed to establish linkages between the health problems of Gulf War veterans and drug, chemical, environmental hazards, other risk factors. That's what the DOD and VA research seems to be showing. At the same time, a growing body of independent research, all peer reviewed—and that's Dr. Moss, Abou-Donia, researchers from the University of Texas, others—continues to find evidence of just such a linkage. Is it that the independent researchers are all wrong and the DOD and VA researchers are all right? Where am I missing something?

Dr. LASHOF. Where I think you're not completely clear on is the kind of research we looked at. We did not look at just what DOD research was or VA research. We reviewed a whole body of research way before—

Senator ROCKEFELLER. That wasn't my question. I understand that you did. But isn't it interesting that DOD and VA say no, the linkages aren't there, it must be something else, i.e., we point to stress, while the independent research does hint at, even though not perfectly proven yet so far, causation or linkages.

Dr. LASHOF. What I was trying to say, Senator, is that not all independent research goes in that direction. The research of Abou-Donia we did review thoroughly. We found it not applicable to this situation because what he did was he used pyridostigmine bromide and DEET at very high doses, much higher than our troops would be exposed to proportionally, recognizing he's dealing with chickens of course, and then he sacrificed them immediately and looked for changes. What we're talking about here in the troops is that they were exposed at one point and then a long time later after they are no longer exposed, where the chemicals are out of their body, they are having symptomatology. So we looked for literature that dealt with what happens to people who are exposed to something, stop using it, how is it metabolized in the body, what can you expect the body to do.

We reviewed a whole body of scientific literature that deals with these kinds of issues unrelated to the specifics of the Gulf War. Pyridostigmine bromide has been used in the treatment of myasthenia gravis for a long time. We know a lot about its metabolism. I'm not saying pyridostigmine bromide and pesticides couldn't be a contributor. We asked for more research specifically around that because we don't think the appropriate research has been done. We do not find the Abou-Donia convincing because of the type of research. But we in no way limited ourselves to DOD and VA-funded research. There's a whole body of peer reviewed research done by lots of independent people on many of these issues over the years.

Senator ROCKEFELLER. Mr. Chairman, my time is way over, but could I just comment. Myasthenia gravis and PB—I understand that.

But let's also be very clear, for public purposes, that larger doses that can be used for those who are sick may have terrible effects on those who aren't.

Dr. LASHOF. Oh, sure.

Senator ROCKEFELLER. It's like when you give insulin to somebody who needs it, it's fine. If you give the same amount of insulin to somebody who doesn't have diabetes, they may die from it.

Dr. LASHOF. Very true. What I was saying is but from the use of larger amounts we understand the metabolism of that drug, what it does to the body. I know what insulin will do to a normal person who has normal insulin and I know how we can use it and what will happen if I use it in a sick diabetic versus a nondiabetic. So we know a lot about pyridostigmine and how you could expect it to act and what you would expect to happen to an individual who was given it.

Senator ROCKEFELLER. Did you know about General Schwarzkopf's XO logs?

Dr. LASHOF. No. No, we did not.

Senator ROCKEFELLER. Thank you.

Chairman SPECTER. Thank you very much, Senator Rockefeller. Senator Jeffords.

Senator JEFFORDS. Thank you, Mr. Chairman. I certainly want to praise you for this hearing as well as Senator Rockefeller for the time he spent in his reign as chairman on this Committee looking into the Gulf War Syndrome. I have a statement I would like to make part of the record.

Chairman SPECTER. Without objection, it will be made a part of the record in full.

[The prepared statement of Senator Jeffords appears on page 51.]

Senator JEFFORDS. I would like to take a look at what this Committee has to do in view of the evidence. Right now, we have a standard that for diseases which may be connected, those that were affected were treated. The question left to us is whether they are entitled to compensation. The area that I have some concern about is with respect to the descendants. We have legislatively taken care of those who, from Agent Orange, have spina bifida. What would your view be with respect to those kinds of diseases that may be carried on? Should we have a presumption of treatment for those other than spina bifida?

Dr. LASHOF. We as a committee did not look into the compensation issue. This was beyond our scope. But I do think that it is essential that we determine whether there is a relationship between any of the exposures our veterans had and any of the defects seen. We looked at that issue as an issue unrelated to compensation per se.

Senator JEFFORDS. Right. I understand that.

Dr. LASHOF. We found that it is very unlikely, given the kinds of chemicals they were exposed to and what we know about sperm and metabolism, mutagenesis and teratogenesis, that the congenital defects seen were due to Gulf War exposures. Studies to date show no linkage. However, there are other major epidemiologic studies around this specific issue that are being pursued and they should give us additional answers. So, at this point, I don't think we can presume anything.

Senator JEFFORDS. It's not a matter of presumption. In the case of the veterans themselves, if there was any likelihood or possibility, they were entitled to treatment, but not to compensation. I don't want to get into the compensation aspect. But we have not established the same standard for the children of veterans as to treatment. Should we?

Dr. LASHOF. I think we have said that there needs to be a look at and treatment should be given for any reproductive problems that are shown to be related. Research to date has not shown that there are any reproductive problems that are related to service at this point. As I say, the studies are ongoing. But we do think reproductive health care should be included in the range of things that are available.

Senator JEFFORDS. That leaves us in a dilemma about the people who need the treatment and who should pay for it.

Dr. LASHOF. As an aside, may I say that if you're looking at extending health insurance and thinking about doing it for children, maybe you should do it for veterans until we get to a universal health insurance, if we're going to go that way in stages.

Senator JEFFORDS. Thank you.

Chairman SPECTER. Dr. Lashof, just pursuing for one moment the question which Senator Jeffords has raised about treatment for reproductive problems, you had recommended in your testimony that there be statutory authority to treat veterans—

Dr. LASHOF. Pardon?

Chairman SPECTER. You had recommended in your testimony earlier that there be statutory authority to treat veterans and their families for problems connected with reproduction issues.

Dr. LASHOF. Yes.

Chairman SPECTER. So you think there is a matter there that ought to be addressed, or do you think we need further scientific evidence of a causal connection?

Dr. LASHOF. We think that the principle that spouses and children should be treated for reproductive problems if they are related needs to be established and then you can go ahead and establish whether they're related. But right now, even if you knew they were related, they could not be treated (except for spina bifida for Agent Orange) is my understanding.

Chairman SPECTER. They are not covered by existing laws is what you're saying.

Dr. LASHOF. That was my point. I believe that's correct.

Dr. LANDRIGAN. There is a huge underlying scientific problem here, Mr. Chairman, and that is that of the many thousands of chemicals that are in use and the many that were used in the Gulf theater only a minority have ever been tested for reproductive effects. Indeed, only a minority have ever been tested for other toxic effects. But there are particularly striking gaps in this arena. A few years ago I chaired a committee at the National Academy of Sciences that Senator Leahy requested be convened to look at the long term effects on children of early pesticide exposure. One of the striking findings of that committee was the enormous gap in toxicologic test data. We're just seeing it playing out here as well.

Chairman SPECTER. Okay. Thank you very much, Dr. Lashof, Dr. Landrigan.

Dr. LASHOF. Could I make one final statement about stress, if I may?

Chairman SPECTER. Of course you may.

Dr. LASHOF. I wanted to respond to Senator Rockefeller. I really want to reemphasize, and I don't know how strongly I can emphasize the point, that when we say stress is a contributing factor or a causal factor for some of the veterans we do not mean just psychological, we mean physical as well. We do not believe that it is good for the veterans, good for the citizens of this country, to continue to labor under the impression that stress is a psychological condition and there's organic disease that's different and not related to stress.

One of the major epidemiologic studies going on at our University of California-Berkeley, School of Public Health has been with bus drivers. Very interesting observation. When you have a group of men who were hired to drive busses and you study the blood pressure, they run in the normal range. They have the same number of hypertensive, the same number at different levels. Put them driving a bus for a year. At the end of the year, the number of bus drivers who have high blood pressure is significantly higher than the general population. We believe that is due to stress. We don't believe their high blood pressure is in their head.

Stress has tremendous impact on the body's physical functioning. This is an area we also say generally, not related to the Gulf War, needs a great deal further research. Dr. Hamburg, who, as you know, is the preeminent person, chaired a special meeting of our committee devoted entirely to the questions of what do we know about the physiologic impact of stress on the body, and what more do we need to know. The statements and wording around stress is something that was based very heavily upon that review of what we know about the physical impact of stress, Dr. Hamburg's view of what more we need to do in the way of research. We would like people to understand we don't think it's in their head.

Senator ROCKEFELLER. I understand, Dr. Lashof. The reason that I emphasize that is I think that is part of the problem when the word "stress" comes out to the American public and, most importantly, to the Persian Gulf veterans affected. In traditional wars you come home and an arm is missing, you're wounded, you're heavily bandaged, and people immediately understand something is wrong and no questions are asked. But when people are talking about stress, they don't think about the bus driver and the deep studies being done at the University of California, they think that somehow it's a kind of "take a pill and go home" type of treatment. And that's the way the veterans feel about it. They feel that what is real to them is being put up as being in the mind by others. That's the reason why I regret that.

Dr. LASHOF. We regret that as well and that is one of the reasons we have put heavy emphasis on the importance of good risk communication. We think the veterans and the rest of the public need to understand a lot more about stress. We will continue to work on that. One of the things I do as associate chair of the Berkeley Wellness Letter is we deal with that kind of thing trying to get the lay community to understand very complicated, sophisticated medical issues.

Chairman SPECTER. Dr. Lashof, we thank you very much. Dr. Landrigan, we thank you.

Dr. LASHOF. Thank you. We appreciate the opportunity.

Chairman SPECTER. That concludes the hearing.

[Whereupon, at 12:10 p.m., the Committee was adjourned, to reconvene at the call of the Chair.]

APPENDIX

PREPARED STATEMENT OF CHAIRMAN ARLEN SPECTER

Good morning. I am pleased to welcome our witnesses to today's hearing on Persian Gulf War syndrome. Before I introduce them, I want to welcome back our members and say to them that I look forward to working with them in this, the 105th Congress.

Today's hearing, which is the first of a series on this issue, will focus on illnesses which plague Persian Gulf War veterans.

It is nearly six years since the Gulf War ended. Yet, more facts such as the Khamisiyah chemical weapons destruction by U.S. military personnel seem to slowly and reluctantly float to the surface like telltale flotsam from a sunken ship. In spite of the best medical researchers in the world, hundreds of studies since 1991 have failed to pinpoint the causes of what is known as Gulf War Syndrome.

We owe it to our veterans not only to provide them the best medical treatment for their symptoms, but equally to determine, if we can, the root causes of their illnesses and why the government—especially the Pentagon—has been slow and inept in uncovering information and investigating this issue. A full public accounting will be a goal of this committee.

To the Committee's Ranking Member, Senator Rockefeller, I want to say that I see an opportunity for the both of us to ensure that our country's veterans receive the very best medical care and services in the world.

We will work together. Senator Rockefeller, would you like to say a few words?

Our witnesses are the Secretary of Veterans Affairs, Mr. Jesse Brown; the acting Director of the Central Intelligence Agency, Mr. George Tenet; and the Chairperson of the Presidential Advisory Committee on Gulf War Veterans' Illnesses, Dr. Joyce Lashof.

I invite the Secretary of Veterans Affairs to begin with his testimony. Thank you.

PREPARED STATEMENT OF SENATOR STROM THURMOND

Mr. Chairman: It is a pleasure to be here today, at the beginning of this new Congress, to continue our review of this matter of great concern. I congratulate you on your selection as chairman of this Committee, and I know you are going to look closely at this issue and all other issues that affect our Nation's veterans. I join you in welcoming our distinguished witnesses, particularly the Honorable Jesse Brown, Secretary of Veterans Affairs; Mr. George Tenet, Acting Director of Central Intelligence; and Doctor Joyce C. Lashof, Chair of the Presidential Advisory Committee on Persian Gulf War Veterans' Illnesses.

The well-being of those who served in the Persian Gulf is an issue that I have vigorously pursued. As chairman of the Armed Services Committee, I have included provisions in Defense authorization bills establishing the Persian Gulf War registry, providing funding for research, and directing a study on low-level exposure to nerve agents.

Mr. Chairman, we learned last year that our troops were exposed to nerve agents released as a result of postwar demolition of chemical rockets at an ammunition storage area in Iraq. In light of these developments, it is critical that the government continue to identify those who may have been exposed to nerve agents to assess their health, and to continue to provide medical care.

I believe both the Department of Veterans Affairs and the Department of Defense are concerned for the well-being of those who served in the Persian Gulf. The Department of Veterans Affairs has taken action to address the many mysteries surrounding the various ailments, commonly described as "Persian Gulf Syndrome." Such actions include the establishment of the Persian Gulf Registry to provide health exams and health monitoring of Veterans, as well as the institution of various research programs to identify the causes of the unexplained illnesses reported by Persian Gulf Veterans.

Mr. Chairman, I thank you for holding this important hearing today. I thank the witnesses for their work on this issue and their testimony today. I look forward to reviewing the testimony of the witnesses and working with you to make sure our veterans are treated fairly and honorably.

PREPARED STATEMENT OF SENATOR JAMES M. JEFFORDS

Chairman Specter, Senator Rockefeller, I would like to thank you for holding these important hearings. I want to communicate to you, Chairman Specter, how much I look forward to working with you on the many issues affecting our nation's veterans.

We gather here again to discuss the disturbing issue of Persian Gulf War Syndrome. Our focus remains on the Department of Veterans' Affairs (VA), the Department of Defense (DoD) and the Central Intelligence Agency (CIA) and their activities in addressing the questions surrounding Persian Gulf War Syndrome. Today I am pleased to be able to consider the determinations of the Presidential Advisory Committee (PAC) in its final report on the research, treatment and overall government response to the health care crisis caused by the conditions and situations veterans were exposed to in the Persian Gulf. This study will help us further narrow the range of possibilities causing symptoms associated with Persian Gulf War Syndrome. Of equal importance, it has identified several problem areas related to the government's role. I continue to be troubled by the treatment by the Department of Defense of personnel documents and information on military operations in the theater, as well as by the PAC's assertion that the DoD did not pursue important leads that could move us closer to the answers we are seeking today.

I found the determinations of the Presidential Advisory Committee to be helpful and very encouraging about the efforts of our government in many areas, including Vets' Centers, which, as many of you know, first began as a pilot program in 1979, in Williston, Vermont. According to the PAC, Vets' Centers "quickly mobilized comprehensive outreach efforts and offered a more targeted and direct approach than subsequent DoD or VA efforts." These Centers have since provided essential services to several hundred thousand veterans and their families who need a helping hand with post-war difficulties. The report has discarded a variety of different theories as to the cause of Gulf War maladies. This is encouraging. However, the report presses that much more needs to be done to further examine remaining possible causal factors, particularly related to the synergistic effects of PB and other risk factors. This issue first caught my attention in 1994 during this Committee's deliberations over chemicals PB and DEET and their effects on personnel when combined with stress. I urge the DoD and VA to accelerate their efforts on research to examine these remaining possible risk factors, or combination of risk factors.

The PAC's conclusions about the DoD's "superficial" response to concerns over chemical and biological exposure of troops is very upsetting. Furthermore, the DoD's choosing to ignore calls from its own Defense Science Board for research on long-term health consequences of low-level exposure to chemical warfare agents is inexcusable. This dismissal of a potentially revealing aspect of Gulf War Syndrome, as well as its categorical insistence for so long that there was no incident of chemical or biological exposure of troops, has severely damaged the reputation of the DoD among the public. Also, I would urge the DoD to change its tune in light of the report's assertion that the DoD lacked responsiveness in developing a thorough pre-deployment health exam of a large sample of troops to ensure better post-deployment medical epidemiology.

One of the few disappointing conclusions I have surmised from the report is that the DoD has not done a good job of incorporating the lessons learned from its past Agent Orange difficulties. The overall lesson being the only way to come to solid conclusions on these matters is to be honest, open and thorough from the beginning. Without the cooperation of the DoD, the VA and other government entities involved cannot do their jobs and the sick veterans and their families must wait, and must suffer. Although the DoD is not represented here today, I intend to make my concerns very clear to the new Secretary and I expect every effort will be made to avoid such future problems.

In conclusion, I do not find joy in criticizing the Department of Defense. However, these criticisms are well-founded and the problems should not be allowed to plague us again. Just as military doctrine teaches our armed forces the most effective use of personnel in a life-threatening military engagement to ensure safety and success, so should it prepare the military for protecting the health of our men and women before, during and after a situation where the possibility of exposure to dangerous chemicals and other risk factors exists. There remain many questions still unanswered about Persian Gulf War Syndrome. I look forward to working with my Congressional colleagues, the departments and the PAC over their extended tenure to answer these questions.

PREPARED STATEMENT OF SENATOR BEN NIGHTHORSE CAMPBELL

I would like to first say congratulations to the VA Committee's new chairman, Senator Specter. I know that the veterans will benefit from his chairmanship. Also, I would like to welcome the newest member of the committee, Senator Hutchinson.

I hope that with the beginning of the 105th Congress, we begin with a new slate regarding the issue of Persian Gulf War illness. I am tired of the old routine where politics, personalities, and blame get the spotlight and the veterans who are now suffering get lost in the shuffle.

Personally, I care less about who is responsible than what should be done to help sick Persian Gulf War veterans. I am less concerned about a single or multiple causes for the illness than I am about treating those veterans who are now ill, which is not to say that finding the cause is not critical.

In the last nine months, this committee has seen this issue resurface, almost daily, which should only remind us that there is still so much work to be done.

I think the Presidential Advisory Commission's report should only lead us to ask more questions in hopes of finding more answers.

Although it is imperative that we continue to examine the cause of this illness, it remains critical that our Persian Gulf War veterans who seek out assistance, receive priority medical care—as is mandated by law.

Although I don't want to diminish the accomplishments made, we should be careful not to trip on our accolades for there is still too much work to be done.

I thank the Chair for holding this hearing today and look forward to the testimony.

PREPARED STATEMENT OF SENATOR LARRY E. CRAIG

Mr. Chairman, I look forward with great interest to reading the testimony on the subject of the Persian Gulf War illnesses. I do, however, want to note for the record, my personal congratulations for our new committee chairman Arlen Specter. His longstanding efforts on the Senate Veterans Affairs Committee are well known, and his energies will be greatly needed as we continue to tackle the difficult veterans issues. Mr. Chairman, I look forward to working with you.

I have been encouraged by the efforts of all departments and agencies involved in dealing with the medical and social issues of the Persian Gulf War illnesses to take a more organized, coordinated, sympathetic and effective approach to the problem. However, we still have a long way to go in addressing all issues. Testimony today will help answer some of our outstanding questions, but we must have evidence based assessments before we can make conclusive findings. These findings are imperative not only to answer the questions of our Gulf War veterans, but to continue strategies necessary to prevent and lessen the likelihood of adverse health outcomes of future deployments. We have a responsibility to give today's and future veterans full disclosure. The government must ensure that veterans have options available to them to seek the help they need.

At this point, I ask that Ms. Debra Smith's (Lewiston, Idaho) letter to the editor of USA Today (12/31/96) be inserted into the record.

[The following letter was submitted for the record.]

USA Today, 12/31/96

Vets battle for help

How can Kathy Elena Jurado, assistant secretary at the Department of Veterans Affairs (VA), even attempt to say the needs of Persian Gulf war veterans and their families have been met ("VA takes complaints seriously," Letters, Thursday)?

As the spouse of an ill gulf war veteran who has battled four years for recognition and treatment of his illnesses, I would like to sit an hour or so with Jurado to review my husband's medical file and documented fight for help.

Upon referral by the local VA medical center, he underwent the comprehensive clinical evaluation protocol for gulf war veterans at the West Los Angeles VA Medical Center in October 1994.

Two years later, he still has not been treated for his diagnosed illnesses, nor has any attempt been made to find a cause of his undiagnosable health problems.

He has been unemployable for two years and has been rated disabled by the Social Security Administration. Yet he does not receive treatment or compensation by the VA.

We recently had to declare bankruptcy due to the inability to pay the medical bills we incurred these past four years.

I can say, as can many others, our needs have not been met. It is time to listen to the masses of veterans and not the single, token spokesperson for an agency no one believes in.

Debra Smith
Lewiston, Idaho

Mr. Chairman, this letter from my constituent paints a disturbing picture of neglect. I am however, pleased to note that since her letter, the VA has contacted the Smith family and they are beginning to receive attention after two years of waiting for treatment and compensation. We understand that Mr. David Smith's records are now under review in Washington DC. After the VA reviews his records, I am confident that he will be given the caring treatment and compensation that he rightfully deserves. I hope that today's activities will be a start in helping resolve other veterans' problems, without them having to write to national publications to get the attention they need.

Mr. Chairman, once again, thank you for scheduling this hearing to let us hear firsthand, more about the findings on Persian Gulf War illnesses. The findings from all of the agencies will help answer the questions of our veterans.

PREPARED STATEMENT OF SENATOR JOHN D. ROCKEFELLER IV

I begin today by congratulating you, Chairman Specter, for your return to the chair of the Senate Committee on Veterans' Affairs. There are many important issues for us to deal with, and I look forward to working together with you in finding solutions to some difficult problems.

I especially want to thank you for calling today's hearing on Persian Gulf War illnesses, and for demonstrating that with you as the new chairman, this committee will show a renewed commitment to the problems confronted by the veterans of the Persian Gulf War.

As most have now come to acknowledge, a large number of previously very healthy men and women returned home from the Persian Gulf with a myriad of health complaints and illnesses. In some cases, they have become greatly disabled. In addition to the pain and losses that our veterans have experienced in coping with these health problems, they also have had to endure the humiliation of initially being told that their problems were not "real." They continue to cope with the fear that they have been exposed to unknown agents with unknown, long-term health consequences. More recently, a number of veterans and active duty military personnel have come forward with accounts of suspected chemical exposures that were confirmed, on site, with the equipment that they had been trained to use; they report how they were told then, and are still being told, "this was not real."

While we have still not been able to uncover the "smoking gun" responsible for these illnesses and health problems, research conducted by those *outside* the DoD and VA, at the Centers for Disease Control, has shown that troops deployed to the Gulf were *three times as likely* as troops deployed elsewhere to suffer fatigue, skin rashes, joint pain, headaches, diarrhea, and memory loss. Yet some continue to insist that because these serious health problems did not require lengthy hospitalizations or result in death, their debilitating consequences for these veterans are somehow not worthy of attention. I continue to reject that type of thinking still bent on proving we don't have a problem.

We have not "done right" by our veterans after they have put themselves at enormous risk to protect our Nation. It is no surprise that they view DoD and the VA with so little credibility. We can and we must do better.

Mr Chairman, I know that you are aware that it is the Department of Defense—not appearing before us today—that continues to have primary responsibility for this issue. I have made it clear that in my view, DoD has not upheld their promise to provide adequate protection for the men and women who volunteered to sacrifice their lives in service to this country.

It now appears that a new, invigorated, and perhaps less biased approach to the DoD investigation *may* be taking hold. But I remain very concerned that the years of poor response by the Pentagon to the problems of these men and women has irrevocably undermined the public's faith in the ability of its government to deal honestly with this issue.

The credibility of DoD has suffered greatly, not only because of this, but also because of other historical and current events, such as the problems of radiation experiments in the 50's, Agent Orange in the 70's, and allegations of sexual crimes and harassment against female military personnel in the 90's.

I realize that there have been recent announcements and developments within DoD to remedy this, and I hope that there will be a clear opportunity to convince me and others that their approach has indeed changed. I look forward to working with you, Mr. Chairman, on exploring ways of putting in place institutional safeguards to prevent the future occurrence of another Persian Gulf War illness, another Agent Orange, another Aberdeen Proving Ground.

I have many concerns and questions about the government's handling of these illnesses, and I will ask our witnesses to address them. They include:

- Why has VA denied almost 95% of the compensation claims for undiagnosed illnesses among Gulf War veterans, very often based on what appears to me to be an arbitrary 2-year time limit?

- Why have years of VA and DoD research investigating possible causes of the Gulf War illnesses proceeded without any attention to the possible chronic effects of exposures to low levels of nerve agents ?
- Why did DoD and the CIA insist that there was no possibility of exposures to chemical agents in the Gulf, despite the existence of a 1991 CIA report describing U.S. demolition of chemical munitions at Khamisiyah?
- Why did the intelligence community—CIA and DoD—fail to deal with the information on Khamisiyah and other possible exposures at the time they occurred? How could this happen? Was this due to some type of interagency rivalry, or simply poor communication?
- Why is it that on one day this week we hear from the President's Advisory Committee that there is simply not enough evidence to support any cause of PGW illness other than stress, but on the very next day, we get word that *independent, peer-reviewed, but non-government research* at the University of Texas again gives strong support to the *possible* linkage of drugs and pesticide and chemical exposures to these illnesses?

One final note before I yield, Mr. Chairman. It is simply outrageous that one individual Senator has stopped America's ratification of the Chemical Weapons Convention treaty which would ban the development, production, possession, or transfer of chemical weapons worldwide. This treaty has the support of the entire civilized world, and would provide critical and immediate protection to our troops. I intend to ask Senator Lott to move this to early consideration in the Senate.

PREPARED STATEMENT OF SENATOR PAUL D. WELLSTONE

Thank you Senator Specter for acting so quickly in calling a hearing on the important issue of Persian Gulf War Illnesses.

Thank you Secretary Brown, Director Tenet and Dr. Lashof for being here to respond to Gulf War veterans' concerns and questions. I think the fact that we are holding this hearing so early in the new Congress reflects not only the importance of this issue among my fellow Senators, but also the tremendous obligation we as a nation have in ensuring that the concerns and needs of our military veterans are addressed.

I recently had the privilege of meeting with a number of Minnesota veterans who bravely served our nation during Operation Desert Shield/Desert Storm. Those courageous Persian Gulf veterans have contacted me in search of answers about what, if any hazardous agents, they were exposed to during the war, why they have returned home from the Persian Gulf feeling sick, and what health care and compensation benefits they are entitled to receive. Those veterans and others like them are complaining about illnesses and symptoms they did not have before the war.

As a member of this committee, I consider myself a veterans' advocate, someone who gives the benefit of the doubt to the veteran and fights hard for their rights to information, compassionate health care, and fair and timely benefits. When Persian Gulf veterans tell me that they are "scared to death" about their health problems, I view it as my personal responsibility and obligation to help them.

On Tuesday of this week, the President announced the results of the final report of the Presidential Advisory Committee on Gulf War Veterans' Illnesses that Dr. Lashof will discuss. I was particularly pleased that they will continue oversight of this issue until at least this fall. I applaud their conclusion that we need to have a thorough investigation of all possible exposures to poisonous gases and other dangerous agents. However, I have some concern that in their findings the advisory panel has singled out *stress* as "likely to be an important contributing factor to the illnesses reported by Gulf War veterans." I want to make sure that in making this assertion that it doesn't become the veteran's "fault" for his or her condition. Clearly, there is much ambiguity as to the source and treatment of Gulf illnesses -- I think in this case we must err on the side of the veterans.

The Department of Defense's belated disclosure that U.S. troops destroyed a bunker containing chemical weapons in southern Iraq, releasing contaminants into the air and possibly exposing over 20,000 American military personnel, combined with the Pentagon's on-going investigation into other possible similar incidents involving chemical or biological weapons has raised additional questions and concerns about the health-related problems of Persian Gulf veterans. As such, I share the report's grave concern about the Pentagon's handling of reported exposures to chemical warfare agents. Furthermore, I support the American Legion's proposal for a congressionally appointed commission to investigate the Department of Defense's handling of this matter.

Is it any wonder that our Persian Gulf veterans question the Pentagon's credibility on this issue and strongly suspect a cover up? Whether it's a coverup, incompetence or some combination of the two, the fact is that the Pentagon's credibility on this issue has been damaged and that is a serious problem. Having said that, I do not want to prolong any suffering by our veterans because of a political sideshow or Pentagon bashing exercise. We need to get on with the business of getting to the bottom of these illnesses and taking care of the needs of our veterans.

Persian Gulf veterans cannot be kept in limbo waiting for the completion of research that should have begun years ago but is just starting now on the health effects of low-level exposures to chemical and other agents. The reasons for this delay are the Pentagon's contention for over five years that there were no chemical exposures and that, in any case, low-level exposures had no effects on health. The fact is there have been few scientific studies of low-level exposures so that no one really knows whether such exposures have long-term health effects.

Whether the issue is Post-Traumatic Stress Disorder, radiation exposure, or Agent Orange, I have had the best teachers in the world -- Minnesota veterans who have suffered from these heart-rending and serious conditions. I'm counting on Minnesota Persian Gulf veterans and their families and others from around the country to continue to educate me about their experiences in the Persian Gulf and their health and other problems since returning home.

Almost every day we hear on TV or read in the papers new reports of chemical and other toxic exposures during the Gulf War. Some reports are contradictory and add to our concern and confusion about exactly what happened during the war. To make matters worse, the Pentagon's record of providing information on the toxic agents exposure has been poor and inadequate.

Along those lines, I was pleased to hear that Secretary Brown may consider extending the presumptive period from its current level of two years for veterans seeking compensation for symptoms related to or associated with their Persian Gulf War service. Obviously, there is still much to learn about these illnesses.

While this and other research is being completed, Persian Gulf veterans who have developed health problems that could be related to their war-time service must be given full access to VA health care and be fairly compensated for disabilities.

We are fortunate to have excellent VA facilities in my state of Minnesota. I have worked with them in the past to ensure that veterans with Post-Traumatic Stress Disorder and diseases linked to agent orange and radiation exposures receive the best care possible. I am confident that the VA and DoD officials here and in Minnesota will work closely with me to see to it that Persian Gulf veterans receive the best medical care, benefits, and services available. I am committed to doing whatever it takes to ensure that our veterans are treated fairly.

Mr. Secretary, Director Tenet, Dr. Lashof—I look forward to hearing your testimony on this issue.

PREPARED STATEMENT OF SENATOR PATTY MURRAY

Mr. Chairman, I want to commend you for convening today's hearing. This is one of the first hearings of the 105th Congress, and appropriately, it should send a message to all veterans of the seriousness with which we all view the Gulf War Syndrome issues and the activist role that I hope this committee will play for the next two years.

Chairman Specter, I join all of my colleagues here on the panel in welcoming you as the Chair of the Committee. It is a new day for the Committee and, I am anxious to work closely with you and your staff as well as continue working with Senator Rockefeller and the staff on our side. I also want to welcome Senator Hutchinson to the Committee and pass to him the title of "newest Committee member." Knowing of your previous service on the House Veterans Affairs Committee, I am sure you will quickly assert yourself here.

And I'd be remiss if I did not welcome back to the Committee my friend Jesse Brown, the Secretary of Veterans Affairs. I know the veterans of Washington state share my delight that you will continue to serve just as you have for most of your adult life; as a passionate and tireless veterans advocate. Mr. Secretary, I look forward to working closely with you and the Department in this Congress.

Today's hearing is the first of many on this important issue. Certainly, we all want to better understand why our Persian Gulf vets are suffering a variety of unexplained illnesses. While I am pleased that more federal resources at the VA, and throughout the government, are being dedicated to these mysterious illnesses, I share the frustration that many feel about the current understanding of Gulf War Syndrome. It has been nearly six years and we have largely failed to provide the necessary answers to our vets and the public about the causes of illnesses associated with service in the Gulf.

My own priority on this issue is to ensure that we are doing all we can to take care of the veterans with health problems. Treat now, ask questions later. We have a responsibility to look after those who risked the ultimate sacrifice in the Gulf. This committee has numerous oversight responsibilities when considering Gulf War Syndrome. Certainly, we must make public all relevant information about chemical exposure, releases and any information that might help us better understand the mysterious illnesses . But in the process, let's not overlook our primary responsibility; the care and treatment of our veterans, some 60,000 of whom are having health problems today.

The Veterans Affairs Committee must also follow closely the nearly 80 studies now underway on Gulf War Syndrome and its potential causes. These research projects must be free from government and political interference; the Committee must be a catalyst for the successful completion of these research projects.

With the release of the Presidential Advisory Committee's report on Gulf War Veterans' Illnesses and continued new revelations from the government, this issue is in the national spotlight. As I traveled around Washington state prior to the beginning of the Congress, my constituents raised this issue with me again and again. We have a significant military presence in Washington state; including thousands of veterans and active duty personnel who served in the Gulf conflict.

One event troubled me greatly and I wish to share it with the Committee to demonstrate why we must be vigilant in our search for information to give the public. One group with ties to the white supremist movement spent more than $20,000 promoting an event including radio and television advertisements and more than 100,000 mailed invitations. Several hundred residents, including many former soldiers, attended the event at which this group claimed the Persian Gulf Syndrome was a communicable disease transmitted through perspiration, blood transfusions, and sexual contact. The only way to refute those who would seek to confuse veterans is through public discourse and disclosure of all relevant information. That's what this Committee must stand for. We cannot let this issue become another tool to divide and confuse the public and vets with health problems.

The release of the Presidential Advisory Committee's Report on Gulf War Veterans' Illnesses provides us with another opportunity to communicate with the public. I commend the President for convening the panel, and I support his call to extend the work of the Advisory Committee for nine additional months. I am particularly pleased that the President has indicated his support for allowing Persian Gulf vets more time to submit disability claims. In most cases the two-year rule works, in this case it clearly does not. I know the President's support for this extension is a direct result of the Committee's hard work and the input of Secretary Brown.

At the same time, I am a little amazed at the PAC report's apparent insistence that stress may prove to be the most likely explanation of Gulf War Syndrome. I do hope all of the panelists here today will devote some attention to this point. I am not a medical doctor but I do suspect that solely blaming stress for Gulf War Syndrome says more about our failure to understand gulf-related illnesses than an actual diagnosis. And I know the public and certainly the vets who have spoken to me about this issue are not ready to accept a diagnosis of stress as the cause of Gulf War Syndrome illnesses.

41-207 97 - 3

The Executive Summary of the PAC report states, "The Government has a significant amount of ground to recover with Gulf War Veterans and the American public, who have come to question whether a lack of data—on possible chemical warfare agent exposures, on the pre- or post-deployment health of veterans, or on the location of troops in theater—indicates a lack of commitment to veterans health." Mr. Chairman, that's where we start this hearing. Let's move forward with the ultimate objectives of providing all care required by those who served as well as making public absolutely all relevant information about Gulf War Syndrome.

Chairman Specter, thank you again for convening this hearing.

PREPARED STATEMENT OF HON. JESSE BROWN, SECRETARY, DEPARTMENT OF VETERANS AFFAIRS

Introduction

Mr. Chairman, I want to congratulate you as you take over the Chair of this Committee. You may be new to this Chair, but your sensitivity to all veterans, and your advocacy for those who served in the Persian Gulf, are well known. It is also good to see you, Senator Rockefeller, a powerful supporter of veterans.

Clearly, we face many challenges in pursuing our mutual goal of serving veterans and their families. Some issues, such as the one we are here to discuss today, are very complex. That is why I am so pleased that this key Committee will have knowledgeable and effective leadership during the 105th Congress.

With that, Mr. Chairman, let me thank you and the Members of the Committee for the opportunity to discuss how VA is meeting the needs of Persian Gulf veterans. At this time, I will briefly summarize these activities,

including our response to the possibility of low-level exposure to chemical warfare agents.

To put this information into perspective, we recall that some media reports glamorized the war as "40 days and nights of thunder" in the air action and "100 hours of lightning ground combat." The rest of the story was not so appealing. Nearly 700,000 U.S. troops spent several months in a harsh, desert environment.

Our warriors were exposed to anxious months of preparations for war, with deep concerns about land mines, chemical and biological warfare attacks, and a well-armed enemy.

They faced stressful combat conditions, smoke from oil fires, infectious parasites, vaccines and drugs to counter the effects of nerve gas, insecticides, toxic petroleum products, depleted uranium, and chemical agents.

When victory was declared, some of our servicemen and women found that their war was not over. Soon after returning from the Gulf, some veterans began to report a variety of symptoms and illnesses. They were suffering from fatigue, memory loss, painful joints, and other physical and psychological problems.

At that time, as an official of the Disabled American Veterans, I added my voice to those calling on the government to look into this matter. We remembered the frustrations of Vietnam veterans waiting for a response to concerns about Agent Orange. We in the veterans community were determined that history should not repeat itself.

When I became Secretary for Veterans Affairs in January of 1993, I was briefed on the actions VA had taken for Persian Gulf veterans. A Persian Gulf Registry, with a special medical examination, had been established even before many of these veterans were released from active duty. (Developed April 18, 1991)

This was a good, early response. But we immediately strengthened it, making this issue one of VA's top priorities.

- We requested and received legislation to give Persian Gulf veterans special eligibility for VA medical care (Public Law 103–210, December 20, 1993).
- We established four Persian Gulf Referral Centers in Birmingham, Houston, Los Angeles and Washington, DC.
- We named an Expert Scientific Advisory Committee, with representatives from our veterans service organizations on it.
- We started an extensive research program including 3 Environmental Hazards Research Centers in Boston, East Orange, NJ and Portland.
- We conducted nationwide clinical training for the staff caring for Persian Gulf veterans.
- We consolidated Persian Gulf benefits claims, to ensure consistent and fair ratings (VA first centralized claims at the Louisville VARO; then added Nashville, Philadelphia and Phoenix.)
- And, we supported legislation to compensate Persian Gulf veterans with undiagnosed illnesses. I wrote to every member of Congress, endorsing this legislation. When the legislation was enacted, we moved quickly to begin paying this compensation (Public Law 103–446, November 2, 1994).

As you know, Mr. Chairman, this law specifies that veterans must have symptoms within a presumptive period, now set at two years, after they left the Persian Gulf. I am very concerned that some claims were denied because the veterans' symptoms did not appear until after the two-year presumptive period.

I wrote to the President to propose that the current presumptive period be reconsidered. I am pleased that earlier this week the President announced he has accepted this proposal, and I am charged with reporting back to him in 60 days regarding extending the limit. I will consult with veterans organizations, Members of Congress, and other interested parties before making my decision.

When the compensation law was passed, we contacted Persian Gulf veterans who had VA Registry examinations, and we invited them to file a claim. We immediately began reviewing claims based on environmental hazards that had been disallowed.

We all know that the questions about health effects of Persian Gulf service can be answered only through research. The President has designated me to take the lead in coordinating all federally sponsored research.

More than 80 Persian Gulf-related research projects are in progress, and others have been completed. Larger VA studies include a long-term mortality study of Persian Gulf veterans, and a national health survey of these veterans and their families. In addition, last year VA established a fourth Environmental Hazards Research Center to study the possibility of reproductive problems related to military service.

We are proud that nearly half of all Persian Gulf research is being conducted at VA hospitals and our affiliated medical schools. But we know how important it is to open up scientific review and inquiry to independent, non-government experts.

That is why we have worked hand-in-hand with the Persian Gulf Expert Scientific Panel, the National Academy of Sciences' Institute of Medicine, the National Institutes of Health Panel, the American Institute for Biological Sciences, and the Presidential Advisory Committee on Gulf War Veterans' Illnesses. And it is why we also have supported research by non-government scientists.

Following DoD's announcement in June 1996 that U.S. troops may have been exposed to chemical warfare agents in the Persian Gulf we moved aggressively to evaluate this information. The available scientific literature suggests that long-term, chronic health problems do not result from exposures that were not marked by acute clinical signs and symptoms.

However, research in this area is limited. We cannot conclude that low-level exposures do not have long-term effects, especially when combined with other environmental factors. More research is needed.

Accordingly, the Persian Gulf Veterans Coordinating Board requested and received funding for three new basic science research projects at $2.5 million, and published a request for proposals in the Commerce Business Daily for studies on low-level exposure to these chemicals.

Mr. Chairman, I have outlined a pattern of forthright and thorough response to the problems reported by our Persian Gulf veterans.

VA is examining Persian Gulf veterans:

- 62,000 have completed Registry examinations; and
- all reported symptoms have been treated seriously and received appropriate medical evaluations.

We are treating Persian Gulf veterans:

- They have made 187,000 outpatient visits;
- there have been 19,000 hospital stays; and
- 74,000 have been counseled at Vet Centers.

VA is working to compensate Persian Gulf veterans:

- 44,000 outreach letters have gone to these veterans informing them of new entitlements (the veterans service organizations helped us in that effort);
- we are reviewing 11,000 cases to ensure proper claims development and adjudication; and
- 27,000 Gulf War veterans are receiving benefits for service-connected disabilities.

And we continue to search for answers:

- We are funding government and independent studies; and
- remaining open to suggestions, from all concerned, for further research.

I have said, on many occasions, "If anyone believes we should be doing something that we are not doing, we want to hear from you." In light of this, I am surprised at some of the criticism I have heard. It has been suggested, for example, that VA has not listened to veterans who reported they had been exposed to chemical warfare agents in the Persian Gulf.

The record shows that VA acted responsibly and aggressively. I have described our actions following DoD's recent disclosure about the demolition of chemical agents in southern Iraq. But VA's record goes back much further.

In 1993, three years prior to the DoD disclosure, VA designed a special clinical protocol. It was meant to detect symptoms related to possible nerve gas exposures.

On November 1, 1993, we responded to a specific group of veterans who thought they had been exposed to chemical warfare agents. We selected the Birmingham VA Medical Center to intensively review the scientific literature on the effects of these chemicals. They developed a specialized neurological examination to look for these effects. This facility continues to serve as a focal point for referral patients including those with chemical agent exposures.

On November 16, 1993, I testified before this Committee, noting that some outside VA would dismiss concerns over chemical warfare agents. I said at that time "VA has a responsibility to remain sensitive to the concerns of veterans. So we have had an open mind from the beginning. Our search for answers has never ruled out chemical agents."

And in the Spring 1994, we revised the Registry questionnaire and code sheet to ask veterans if they believed they were exposed to chemical warfare agents.

These activities continue to be important, and they are being carried out today in VA medical facilities nationwide.

There is one other area in which I would like to set the record straight. Some recent media accounts implied that VA was discharging physicians on the basis of their comments or activities relating to Persian Gulf veterans. These allegations are totally false. If VA employees were fired for advocating the cause of veterans, then I would be the first one out the door. I have spent my entire career as an advocate for veterans and as Secretary for Veterans Affairs that has not changed.

As you know, Mr. Chairman, in order to make the fullest use of available resources, VA has had to reduce staff. Any reductions which have occurred, or which will take place, are based on an assessment of staffing and budget requirements. The two physicians who have received the most media attention regarding staff reductions are a part-time doctor and a trainee on a one-year fellowship.

Running the nation's largest health care system is clearly a big management challenge. Balancing budget requirements with the need for sensitivity is never easy. But I believe most VA employees feel, as I do, that Persian Gulf veterans are not faceless statistics. They are individual American citizens who answered their country's call and served bravely. They are individuals who come to us with genuine problems and concerns for their future.

We are absolutely committed to responding to those problems and concerns with efficiency and compassion. And I repeat once again my open invitation to this Committee and others in the Congress to let us have your recommendations. We will always welcome and fully consider all viewpoints in this critically important area.

Health Care and Research Programs

Shortly after returning from the Persian Gulf War, some veterans began to report a variety of symptoms and illnesses. In preparation for the expected needs of our latest combat veterans, VA immediately began development of its Persian Gulf programs. The first component of the VA's comprehensive Gulf War response was the establishment of a health-care program, the VA Persian Gulf Registry health examination program. The Registry was developed in 1991 and implemented in 1992. Persian Gulf health programs in the early days after the war were already being given high priority and attention. In 1993, at the request of VA, Congress enacted Public Law 103–210, giving Persian Gulf veterans special eligibility for VA health care.

VA's Persian Gulf programs are encompassed in a comprehensive four-pronged approach, addressing relevant medical care, research, compensation, and outreach and educational issues. VA provides Persian Gulf Registry health examinations and follow-up care at its medical facilities nationwide, specialized evaluations at four regional Referral Centers, and readjustment and sexual trauma counseling to Persian Gulf War veterans. To date, more than 63,000 Persian Gulf War veterans have completed Registry examinations, almost 187,000 have been seen in VA ambulatory care clinics, more than 19,000 have been hospitalized at VA medical facilities, more than 350 veterans have received specialized Referral Center evaluations, and more than 74,000 have been counseled at VA's Vet Centers.

Persian Gulf veterans participating in the Registry examination program have commonly reported that they suffer from a diverse array of symptoms including fatigue, skin rash, headache, muscle and joint pain, memory problems, shortness of breath, sleep disturbances, gastrointestinal symptoms, and chest pain. These symptoms have been treated seriously and they have received appropriate medical evaluations. To date, the diagnoses received by Registry participants do not cluster in one organ system or disease category, but rather span a wide range of illnesses and diagnostic categories. As such, they do not meet the clinical definition of a medical syndrome per se. Having said this, though, in no way diminishes how we view these complaints or what type of evaluation the symptomatic person receives. Also of particular note, 12 percent of the VA Registry examination participants have had no current health complaints but have wished to participate in the examination because they were concerned that their future health might be affected as a consequence of their service in the

Persian Gulf War. While 26 percent of the Registry participants rated their health as poor, 73 percent receiving this examination reported their health as all right to good.

With regard to the possible troop exposure to chemical warfare nerve agents, the Department of Defense has provided VA with a list of 21,799 individuals who they identified likely being present within 50 kilometers of the Khamisiyah Ammunition Storage Area during the demolition period in March 1991. A computer match of the Persian Gulf Health Examination Registry database with this list identified 1,978 veterans, or approximately 9 percent, had completed Registry examinations prior to September 1996. A comparison of the examination results of these individuals with other Registry participants shows that similar types and rates of symptoms, diagnoses, and self-reported health status are reported, but virtually no individual in this group reported no symptoms at the time of their Registry examinations. Furthermore, those Registry participants (n=81) who are identified as part of the on-site Khamisiyah demolition team report symptoms and are diagnosed with musculoskeletal conditions at a higher rate than the 50 kilometer or general Registry group. This health surveillance data is preliminary and is compiled from evaluations of a self-selected group of the individuals possibly exposed to nerve agents at Khamisiyah. The results should not be generalized to the entire Khamisiyah group or considered definitive. A copy of this compiled clinical data as been provided to the Committee.

At this point, I should also note that the Persian Gulf Registry was never intended or designed to be a scientific study. It is a health-care program which was established to assist veterans' entry into the continuum of VA care. As such, we encourage all Persian Gulf War veterans, symptomatic or not, to get a Registry examination. Furthermore, if Persian Gulf War veterans have health problems that may be related to an exposure that occurred during their Gulf service, they are eligible for outpatient and inpatient care at VA medical facilities.

While some symptoms of Persian Gulf veterans are difficult to diagnose and remain unexplained, there is consensus among government and non-government physicians and scientists that current evidence does not support the existence of a single unique Persian Gulf Syndrome. The results of recently published research studies also has indicated that Persian Gulf veterans are not suffering at higher rates from life-threatening medical conditions or being hospitalized at higher rates than their non-deployed counterparts. Does this mean that there is no problem and that Persian Gulf veterans concerns are being dismissed or ignored by VA? The answer is an emphatic no.

Statements about the lack of a Gulf War Syndrome should not be misconstrued as being equivalent to a denial of the pain, concerns and complaints of Persian Gulf veterans. Persian Gulf veterans who seek care from VA are suffering from genuine illnesses and, as indicated already, we are providing treatment for these persons. Likewise, VA provides compensation for many of those who are disabled and is conducting research programs to better understand the nature and causes for their illnesses.

The record shows that VA has always acknowledged the possibility that Persian Gulf War veterans were exposed to a wide variety of hazardous agents while serving in the Southwest Asia theater of operations, including chemical warfare agents. VA's public statements have always been clear that all exposures, including chemical warfare agents, were being investigated. In 1993, VA designed its clinical uniform case assessment protocol to detect clinical signs and symptoms related to possible nerve gas and other neurotoxic exposures. Neurologic examinations and cognitive testing were part of the earliest versions of this protocol. As a consequence, VA diagnostic protocols continue to serve as a valid set of clinical guidelines for initial screening examinations (Phase I) and more comprehensive evaluations of difficult-to-diagnose cases (Phase II). These protocols received positive reviews by highly-respected physicians and scientists in the past, and they will be reviewed once more later this year by a newly constituted Institute of Medicine Committee. To date, no valid diagnostic test has been found to identify chemical warfare agent exposures that occurred years ago; therefore, no confirmatory test can be performed for veterans who wish to know whether or not they were exposed to these toxins during their service in the Gulf. Unfortunately, the protocol cannot be revised to make this assessment because the technology simply does not exist.

In the wake of the recent information regarding release of nerve agents at Khamisiyah in March 1991, VA has been asked whether we listened to veterans who reported their belief that they had been exposed to chemical warfare agents during their Persian Gulf service. We believe that there is undeniable evidence that VA officials did listen to those veterans and did take appropriate action to investigate their concerns. As an example, members of a Navy Reserve Construction Battalion unit from Alabama, Tennessee, North Carolina, and Georgia reported suffering adverse health effects which they attributed to exposure to chemical warfare agents during their Persian Gulf War service. In response, VA established a pilot medical program at the Birmingham VA Medical Center to evaluate their health status. As part of this special health-care program, more than 100 veterans were evaluated and treated. Veterans with cognitive symptoms received extensive (7–8 hour) neuropsychological testing and clinical evaluations.

Furthermore, the VA revised Registry examination protocol routinely asks participants to report the exposures they believe occurred during their service in Desert Shield and Desert Storm, including possible exposure to mustard gas or nerve agents. VA's openness to veterans views and concerns is also evident in the representation of veteran service organizations on the VA Persian Gulf War Expert Scientific Advisory Committee. In addition to these clinical programs, research studies are underway to investigate the prevalence of symptoms and medical conditions among Gulf War veterans and to determine whether they are associated with the wide range of reported risk factors, including chemical warfare agents.

In order to get the best assessment of the health status of the veterans, a carefully designed and well-executed research program is necessary. VA, as lead agent for federally sponsored Persian Gulf War research programs, has already laid the foundation for such a research plan. Under the auspices of the Persian Gulf Veterans Coordinating Board's Research Working Group, VA has developed a structured research portfolio to address the currently recognized, highest priority medical and scientific issues. More than 80 research projects are in progress and others have been completed. We continue to search for answers and to expand our understanding of the complex array of issues related to Persian Gulf War veterans' illnesses. While scientific answers are being sought, VA also continues to provide Persian Gulf War veterans with needed health care and other services to reduce their suffering.

VA's own research programs related to Persian Gulf veterans' illnesses include more than 30 individual projects being carried out nationwide by VA and University-affiliated investigators.

VA established three Environmental Hazards Research Centers in 1994. All three centers are carrying out projects which address aspects of the potential adverse health outcomes of exposure to a wide variety of hazards, including neurotoxins. In 1996, we established a fourth center at the Louisville VAMC for investigation of adverse reproductive outcomes. In addition, VA's Environmental Epidemiology Service has completed an initial Persian Gulf Veterans Mortality Study and has begun a long-term mortality study. The VA National Health Survey of Persian Gulf Veterans and Their Families is being carried out by the VA's Environmental Epidemiology Service. Phase I, a postal survey of 15,000 Gulf War veterans and a comparison group of 15,000 Gulf era veterans, was completed in August 1996. The questions on this survey asked veterans to report health complaints, medical conditions, and possible exposures to a wide variety of possible environmental agents, including potential nerve gas or mustard gas exposure. The response rate for Phase I of this postal survey was good, with an adjusted response rate of approximately 57 percent. Phase II will consist of 8,000 telephone interviews and a review of 4,000 medical records. Phase II will address the potential for non-response bias, provide a more stable estimate of prevalence rates for various health outcomes, and verify self-reported health outcomes in medical records. The Phase III examination protocol is being finalized and examinations of veterans and their family members are expected to begin in Spring 1997. Peer-review is provided by a subcommittee of VA's Persian Gulf War Expert Scientific Advisory Committee. Details of these and other government-sponsored research studies are included in the report, *Federally Sponsored Research on Persian Gulf Veterans Illnesses for 1995*. Copies of this report have been provided to the Committee.

In January 1994, the President established the Persian Gulf Veterans Coordinating Board, chaired by the Secretaries of VA, DoD, and HHS, to provide interdepartmental coordination and direction of federal programs related to Persian Gulf War veterans. The Coordinating Board provides an interdepartmental means to share information on Persian Gulf War veterans health, to allocate available resources to the apparent highest priorities, and to disseminate new research information. The Coordinating Board has three specific objectives:

- to ensure that all veterans are provided the complete range of healthcare services necessary to take care of medical problems that may be related to deployment in Operations Desert Shield and Desert Storm;
- to develop a research program that will result in the most accurate and complete understanding of the health problems experienced by Persian Gulf War veterans and the factors that have contributed to these problems; and
- to develop clear and consistent guidelines for the evaluation and compensation of disabilities related to Persian Gulf service.

VA plays a central role in the Persian Gulf Veterans Coordinating Board through its participation in the Clinical, Research, and Compensation and Benefits Working Groups. In particular, the Research Working Group provides guidance and coordination for VA, DoD and HHS research activities related to Persian Gulf War veterans' health. It coordinates all studies conducted or sponsored by these three departments in order to prevent unnecessary duplication and to ensure that important gaps in scientific knowledge are identified and addressed. The working group is actively involved in directing resources toward high priority questions and monitoring the results of federally sponsored research projects. It has produced two reports: the *Report of Federal Research Activities Related to Persian Gulf Veterans Illnesses* and the 1996 update of *A Working Plan for Research On Persian Gulf Veterans Illnesses.*

One example of the Coordinating Board's proactive role in relevant research administration was its prioritization of the federal government and non-government research proposals submitted for funding pursuant to DoD's 1996 Broad Agency Announcement. The American Institute for Biological Sciences (AIBS) performed peer-review of the 111 proposals submitted. The research working group reviewed those proposals judged scientifically meritorious by AIBS and prioritized them according to relevance and potential to fill research gaps in the existing Persian Gulf research portfolio. Twelve research projects encompassing the areas of reproductive outcomes, toxicology of pyridostigmine bromide, modeling of respiratory toxicant exposures from tent heaters, neuropsychological outcomes, immune dysfunction, mycoplasma infection, leishmaniasis, chronic fatigue, fibromyalgia, and neuromuscular function were given high priority for funding by the research working group.

Studies of the potential long-term health effects of low-level (asymptomatic) chemical warfare agent exposure were not given a high priority in the 1995 Working Plan or other research questions because military and intelligence sources had repeatedly stated that there had been no use, presence, or evidence of exposure to chemical warfare agents in the theater of operations. Based on these repeated assertions, combined with a lack of clear-cut clinical evidence to support a finding of chemical warfare exposure, the Coordinating Board focused its research resources on other questions. However, while exposures per se were not a focus of research, clearly the health outcomes which could result from such a neurotoxic exposure were given priority. These outcomes included cognitive, neurologic, and neuromuscular effects. This decision was supported by committee reports from the Institute of Medicine, VA Persian Gulf Expert Scientific Committee, the National Institutes of Health Technology Assessment Workshop, the Presidential Advisory Committee, and others.

When DoD made its June 1996 announcement regarding possible exposure of U.S. troops to sarin and cyclo-sarin as a result of the demolition at Khamisiyah, the Coordinating Board immediately began revision of its action plan. Through the Research Working Group of the Coordinating Board, VA has developed an action plan to address possible long-term health consequences of low-level exposure to chemical warfare nerve toxins and mustard gas.

A recent literature review carried out by independent, non-government and government scientists, suggests that readily-identifiable, long-term adverse health effects due to nerve agent exposures only occur in humans who show signs of acute toxicity or poisoning. However, I should note that the research in this area is sparse and the absence of proof is not proof of absence. In VA's judgment, this information does not mean that clinically important adverse health effects cannot or definitely do not occur in the setting of low-level neurotoxin exposures, especially if combined with other components or environmental stressors. The Coordinating Board has recommended that more research resources be allocated to address this question. I strongly agree with this approach. The Research Working Group has reconsidered the matter and intensified its efforts related to possible effects of low-level exposures to chemical warfare agents.

Based on the Coordinating Board's recommendation, $2.5 million dollars has already been allocated to three new, peer-reviewed, basic science research projects in this area, and an additional $2 million has been identified for additional studies. Funding for these new efforts will come from the DoD/VA collaborative research program that is funded as part of DoD's appropriation. Furthermore, a request for proposals on low-level chemical warfare nerve agent exposures was developed by the Coordinating Board and published in the December issue of the Commerce Business Daily. A copy has been provided to the Committee.

While these efforts represent a good beginning, the Under Secretary for Health has asked VA's Research Service to take a completely fresh look at these issues in light of the new information provided by DoD. This includes asking them to develop a strategic plan for an environmental health research agenda that specifically focuses on low-level exposures to neurotoxins that might result from chemical warfare agents or other military situations. This is due to the Undersecretary in February. Likewise, we are in the process of organizing an international scientific symposium that bridges potential military and civilian incidents involving exposure to those types of chemicals. Given the relative lack of worldwide scientific capability for assessing these issues in the traditional open and peer-reviewed manner in which the best science is carried out, we believe it is essential to bring together a multi-disciplinary group of experts to focus on finding innovative solutions to these perplexing issues.

Research related to the illnesses of Persian Gulf War veterans is highly complex, and this is especially so for the investigation of concerns related to possible low-level exposure to chemical warfare agents. VA is committed to meeting these challenges and obtaining the most accurate answers we can concerning the health of PGW veterans and their families. The recently submitted final report of the

Presidential Advisory Committee on Gulf War Veterans' Illnesses will be particularly useful in this regard.

VA was proactive in establishing health-care programs for Persian Gulf War veterans. In the immediate post-war period, the medical and scientific community had only limited knowledge of the complexity of Gulf War specific issues and exposures. Through our clinical and research programs, VA has been a leader in the development and dissemination of knowledge on Gulf War-related health issues. In order to keep our health-care providers well-informed on the latest developments, VA has utilized a wide array of communication vehicles including periodic nationwide conference calls, mailings, satellite video-teleconferences and annual on-site continuing medical education (CME) conferences. Our initial efforts were successful in educating a dedicated cadre of well-informed Registry physicians and staff, and we will continue to keep them up-to-date on the latest developments. However, I see an opportunity to improve the understanding of Persian Gulf war-related health issues by other medical personnel. My goal is that all VA health-care providers will have a working understanding of Gulf War exposures and health issues and will be able to discuss with their Persian Gulf patients how these issues could impact on their current or future health status. In order to meet this challenge and continue to improve our programs, the Veterans Health Administration has developed and will publish a self-study Persian Gulf CME program for every VA physician in early 1997. We will make this available to non-VA physicians, at cost, as well.

Persian Gulf veterans are not faceless statistics to VA health care personnel. They are individual American citizens who have answered their country's call to arms and served their nation bravely. They are individuals who come to us with genuine problems and concerns for their future. Our doctors, nurses, therapists and directors are dedicated to providing compassionate care, compensation examinations and answering medical question. We will push forward with our programs. If we fall short of the high standards we set for ourselves, we will strive harder to achieve our goal of continuous improvement. President Clinton has made it clear that no effort should be spared in this regard. In the end, long after the headlines fade away and national attention turns elsewhere, VA will still be there to care for Persian Gulf veterans. It is our mission. It is our nation's irrevocable promise to its veterans.

In this regard we are grateful for the assistance provided by the Presidential Advisory Committee on Gulf War Veterans' Illnesses. We recognize the central role they played in investigation of possible troop exposure to sarin and cyclo-sarin. The recommendations released in the Committee's final report will be given serious consideration. As the President has directed, I along with the Secretaries of Defense and

Health and Human Services will be preparing an action plan addressing the Committee's recommendations. This action plan, which will be developed by the Coordinating Board, will be presented to the President within 60 days.

Compensation Programs

After the return of U.S. forces from the Persian Gulf, many veterans began exhibiting symptoms that even today cannot be readily attributed to a known clinical diagnosis. There were concerns that these illnesses were caused by chemical exposure or other environmental hazards in the Persian Gulf. Because of these concerns, the Veterans Benefits Administration (VBA) centralized the adjudication of Persian Gulf compensation claims based on environmental hazards in the Louisville Regional Office, beginning December 1992. In October 1994, we redistributed this responsibility to four regional offices, known as "Area Processing Offices" (APOs), Louisville, Nashville, Phoenix, and Philadelphia. Centralization allowed these offices to gain expertise in the complex issues involved and gave us an opportunity to monitor more easily the processing of these claims.

Since the wide array of symptoms presented by many Persian Gulf veterans continued to defy explanation and diagnosis, we were unable to pay compensation for them under the usual statutory authority, 38 U.S.C. 1110. This provision gives us the authority to compensate for disabilities that arise from diseases or personal injuries incurred or aggravated in the line of duty during active military, naval, or air service. The accepted definition of "disease" includes the notion that it is manifested by a characteristic set of symptoms and signs whose etiology, pathology, and prognosis may be known or unknown. In other words, a "disease" displays certain signs and symptoms that can be attributed to a known clinical diagnosis. This definition excluded the undiagnosed illnesses of Persian Gulf veterans.

Therefore, in a series of hearings held in the summer of 1994, we urgently requested legislation giving us specific authority to compensate for these undiagnosed illnesses. In October 1994, the Congress passed what became Public Law 103–446, signed by the President on November 2. This statute allows us to pay compensation to any Persian Gulf veteran with a chronic disability resulting from an undiagnosed illness or combination of undiagnosed illnesses that appeared either during active duty in the Persian Gulf or to a degree of 10 percent or more within a presumptive period thereafter.

In September 1994, even before the final legislation was formulated, we formed a working group to prepare regulations to implement the statute that we were anticipating. The hard work we put into the rulemaking was successful. On February 3, 1995, barely three months after the President signed Public Law 103–446, we published 38 CFR 3.317 to implement the criteria for establishing service connection for undiagnosed illnesses. In this rule, we established a two-year presumptive period for disabilities resulting from undiagnosed illnesses. Since the presumptive period remains a point of controversy, I would like to take a few moments to explain the rationale for selecting that particular period of time.

Public Law 103–446 required that we establish a presumptive period after taking into account three factors: (1) the credible scientific and medical evidence, (2) the historical treatment afforded disabilities for which manifestation periods have been previously established, and (3) any other pertinent circumstances regarding the experiences of Persian Gulf War veterans.

There is little or no medical or scientific evidence definitively linking the undiagnosed illnesses with service in the Gulf. The evidence supports no conclusions that would justify adopting any particular presumptive period. Therefore, we had to rely on historical treatment and pertinent circumstances.

For many years the statute has authorized a one-year presumptive period for various chronic diseases, many of which present signs and symptoms similar to those of the undiagnosed illnesses of Persian Gulf veterans. However, a one-year period would not have met the particular needs of these veterans, since it was not immediately apparent that their illnesses would present the problems that remain unresolved today. On the other hand, two years following service in the Gulf provided an adequate period of time in which all veterans of the hostilities would have had an opportunity to document health concerns arising after their departure from the Gulf.

As soon as the final regulation was published we issued instructions concerning adjudication of claims under the undiagnosed illness criteria. Between February and August 1995, we mailed outreach letters to 44,292 veterans informing of their potential entitlement to compensation under Public Law 103–446.

We assigned jurisdiction for these claims to the four APOs already handling Persian Gulf compensation claims based on environmental hazards and developed a tracking system for monitoring the cases and for report purposes. Their first task under the new regulation was to review environmental hazard claims in which service connection had been denied.

Since we continued to hear reports that many Persian Gulf veterans were first developing unexplained illnesses well beyond two years after their return from the Gulf, we became concerned about the adequacy of the two-year period. Therefore, between March and May of 1996, VA reviewed a sample of these cases. We found instances where recent medical examinations or lay statements could have proved important to the veterans' claims. We were concerned that these veterans might not have received proper information about the sources of information that they could use to establish the merits of their claims.

On the basis of these findings, in July we instructed the APOs to undertake a readjudication of approximately 11,000 cases to ensure proper claims development and adjudication. To date we have completed review of about 2,100 cases. The readjudication has proved to be a lengthier and more complex undertaking than we had anticipated. I am sure you will agree that the second look we give to these cases must be careful and comprehensive.

But let me focus on the outcomes of Persian Gulf veterans' claims. As of the end of December, we had received compensation claims from 84,147 Persian Gulf veterans and awarded compensation to 27,301 of them, or 32.4 percent. In addition, in recognition that disabilities are present, another 37,700 Persian Gulf veterans have been granted service connection at zero percent. Let me turn now to the more specific subject of undiagnosed illnesses. Bear in mind, first of all, that service connection for an undiagnosed illness is considered only after we attempt to establish service connection on the basis of a diagnosis for that condition. A GAO report issued in May 1996 stated that of the undiagnosed illness cases they reviewed, some 60 percent of the veterans were receiving compensation for diagnosed conditions. Subsequent reviews in VA have validated GAO's findings. These independently derived figures strongly suggest that over 50 percent of Persian Gulf veterans claiming compensation for undiagnosed illnesses are receiving compensation for diagnosed conditions.

In recent months I have received several recommendations from veterans, veterans' service organization, and members of Congress urging me to extend the two-year period. Recommendations have ranged from establishing a five-year period to keeping the period completely open-ended. As you may be aware, Senator Wellstone and Congressman Evans have informed me that they have prepared legislation to extend the presumptive period to ten years. Many proponents of a longer presumptive period point to DOD's disclosures concerning possible exposure to chemical weapons and the uncertainties of science and medicine about the chronic health effects of low-level exposure and conclude that I should give veterans the benefit of the doubt.

I can assure you that we will carefully review the need to extend the presumptive period. That concludes my statement. My colleagues and I would be happy to answer any questions you may have.

PREPARED STATEMENT OF GEORGE J. TENET, ACTING DIRECTOR, CENTRAL INTELLIGENCE AGENCY

Chairman Specter and Members of the Veterans Affairs Committee, I am pleased to appear before you this morning to discuss CIA's efforts on the issue of Gulf War illnesses. I am accompanied today by CIA's Executive Director, Nora Slatkin. I want to emphasize at the outset that we know how important this issue is to Gulf War veterans and that we in the CIA will do whatever we can to help.

To go over the background first, the CIA has focused its energies on the intelligence aspects of this issue.

- We began a comprehensive review of all intelligence reporting in March 1995. We started at this date because of the President's concerns and because of issues raised by CIA employees. Until then, we were focused on uncovering still-hidden elements of Iraq's chemical and biological weapons programs. This work was important to support UNSCOM's effort to eliminate those programs.

- In our review, we examined all the intelligence reporting to help DoD determine whether or not US troops were exposed to chemical or biological agents during the Gulf War. The exposure could have been either through Iraqi use or through destruction of Iraq's chemical or biological facilities.

- We identified Khamisiyah as a potential exposure site in the course of this effort. We then took the initiative to determine what had happened there.

- The Presidential Advisory Committee last spring then asked us to arrange to model events during and after the war resulting in the release of chemical agents into the atmosphere.

- As we told you during a briefing in September, we used a contractor to model releases at Muhammadiyat, Al Muthanna, and Bunker 73 at Khamisiyah.

- We were unable to have the contractor model the pit area destruction at Khamisiyah in March 1991. The data were too uncertain.

After long efforts, we think that everything possible has been done to try to model the chemical release at the Khamisiyah pit. We have learned lessons from our work. We will draw on them in the future.

As for next steps, we will continue to work with DoD and the Presidential Advisory Committee to help get answers on these important issues. We are also prepared to address your questions after this briefing.

Key Findings

Let me now go into our key findings. Since we met with you in September, our basic intelligence assessments remain unchanged. Allow me to briefly summarize those findings.

First, we continue to believe, on the basis of a comprehensive review of intelligence, that Iraq did not deploy chemical or biological weapons in Kuwait or use them during the Gulf War.

Second, analysis and computer modeling indicate chemical agents released by aerial bombing of chemical warfare facilities did not reach US troops in Saudi Arabia.

Finally, our review surfaced evidence that CW agents had been released at two separate locations near Khamisiyah in southern Iraq as a result of US demolition activity.

What is new since our last appearance before you is that we have worked with an Expert Review Group to evaluate the methodologies used in modeling efforts. This is the group requested by then-DCI Deutch and convened by Deputy Secretary of Defense White. John Deutch recognized that the modeling of the demolition activity in the pit area near Khamisiyah was crucial to DoD's efforts to determine possible exposure of US veterans. He wanted to assemble the broadest possible expertise to ensure that the modeling effort was unassailable.

To this end, DoD asked the Institute of Defense Analysis (IDA) to convene a panel drawn from the scientific and technical community. The panel first met in late November and we anticipate its final report shortly for release to the public. CIA briefed the panel on the modeling efforts and shared with it the evidence, assumptions, and methodologies. Although CIA plans to sponsor no further modeling, we will continue to work with DoD as it follows up on IDA's recommendations.

Let me take a moment to review CIA's role in analyzing Iraq's chemical and biological weapons programs to help put into context our participation in investigating US exposure to chemical agents. I will break my remarks into three parts—our intelligence focus before, during, and after the war.

Before the War

The Intelligence Community has long followed Iraq's chemical and biological programs as part of its mission to assess chemical and biological weapons capabilities worldwide. Before the war, CIA, like others in the Intelligence Community, assessed that Iraq had a significant chemical and biological weapons capability, including chemically armed Scuds. We also assessed that Iraq had used chemical weapons on numerous occasions against Iran and its own citizens. The Intelligence Community at the time had reached consensus that Iraq had chemical weapons in its arsenal, had forward-deployed these weapons, and was prepared to use them against coalition forces.

During the War

As Desert Storm began, our concerns about the Iraqi use of weapons of mass destruction became the foremost focus of our chemical and biological weapons analytic and collection efforts. Our analysts, in cooperation with their colleagues in other agencies, sought to identify possible Iraqi CW and BW facilities for targeting purposes. In all, 32 sites were identified, albeit on incomplete and sometimes inaccurate information.

A key objective for both military and intelligence personnel was the early detection of the use of chemical or biological weapons. We received several reports of detection alarms. CIA operated a 24-hour chemical and biological detection unit at the start of the air war and maintained it through the ground campaign to monitor and assess such reports.

After the War

In the months immediately following the Gulf War, we turned our intelligence assets to identifying and characterizing Iraq's CW and BW capabilities. The primary focus of our intelligence efforts during 1993 and 1994 consisted of supporting UNSCOM inspections, assessing Iraq's declarations on issues of weapons of mass destruction, refining collection requirements, and interpreting intelligence to attempt to root out the remaining Iraqi CW capabilities.

During this time CIA also worked with DoD to try to track down and check the validity and possible causes of chemical detections that had occurred during the War. A good example of this was the 19 January 1991 Czech detection of nerve agents in Saudi Arabia. In this case, we sent a detailee to Czechoslovakia to further research the claim. We also had our contractor/modeler look at possible causes for the detections. We concluded that the detections were credible due to the specificity of the equipment and the quality of the procedures used by the Czechs. However, we were unable to conclusively determine the cause. We nonetheless remain convinced that the presence of chemical agents was not due to Iraqi offensive actions such as the use of Scud missiles.

In March 1995, CIA began a thorough reexamination of relevant intelligence. We did so because of the President's expressed concern about Gulf War Illness and because of questions raised by two CIA employees. This review culminated in the publication of our report last August.

During this reexamination, we reviewed thousands of intelligence reports and other intelligence holdings.

CIA analysts drew on information from DoD and other sources to clarify intelligence, get leads, and ensure a comprehensive assessment. Our study complemented DoD investigations that used troop testimony, medical records, and operational logs.

Let me address head-on a question that is probably on your mind, and one we have asked ourselves: why didn't CIA and the Intelligence Community focus on the potential exposure issue earlier? A number of reasons contributed to the gap between 1991 and March 1995, when we began this intelligence review. From the beginning, the consensus within the US Government was that Iraq had not used chemical or biological weapons during the war. Analysis since then has maintained that view. Moreover Iraq engaged in widespread deception with regard to where it stored its chemical weapons. Therefore, many reports received during this time were viewed with skepticism.

Shortly after the war, the conditions-now commonly referred to as Gulf War illness-had not yet been widely reported. CIA's intelligence requirements did not make it a priority to examine all incidents of potential low-level exposure.

In these circumstances, the Intelligence Community remained focused on its mission to support UNSCOM and assess the remaining Iraqi CBW capabilities.

When we did focus more broadly on potential exposures short of actual Iraqi use, we identified two primary scenarios: fallout from aerial bombings in Iraq or fallout from demolition activity in the Kuwaiti Theater of Operation. Let me turn first to fallout from aerial bombings.

Based on currently available information, we conclude that Coalition aerial bombing damaged filled chemical munitions at two facilities—Muhammadiyat and Al Muthanna. Both are located in remote areas west of Baghdad. (See briefing board) Iraq recently claimed that less than 5 percent of its approximately 700 metric tons of chemical agent stockpile was destroyed by Coalition bombing. In most cases, the Iraqis did not store chemical munitions in bunkers that they believed the Coalition would target. They stored many of these munitions in the open to protect them from Coalition detection and bombing. In addition, Iraq had inactivated or dismantled all known CW agent and precursor production lines by the start of the air campaign.

At the request of the Presidential Advisory Committee, CIA had modeling performed of releases from these facilities. That modeling work indicates that fallout from these facilities did not reach troops in Saudi Arabia.

At Muhammadiyat Storage Area, Iraq declared that 200 mustard-filled and 12 sarin-filled aerial bombs were damaged or destroyed by Coalition bombing. Bombing of this facility started on 19 January and continued throughout the air war. Analysis of all available information leads us to conclude that the earliest chemical munitions destruction date at Muhammadiyat is 22 January. We have had models created showing a worst case release of 2.9 metric tons of sarin and 15 metric tons of mustard for all possible bombing dates. For these days, as for the whole time period of the bombing, southerly winds occurred on only a few days. The maximum downwind dispersions in the general southerly direction for sarin and mustard cut off at about 300 and 130 km respectively. Neither the first effects nor the lower exposure levels—known as "general population limit" levels—reached US troops that were stationed in Saudi Arabia.

At Al Muthanna, the primary Iraqi CW production and storage facility, Iraq declared that 2,500 chemical rockets containing about 17 metric tons of sarin nerve agent had been destroyed by Coalition bombing. Analysis of all available information leads us to conclude that the earliest chemical munitions destruction date is 6 February. Of the days that the bunker at Muthanna could have been bombed, winds were southerly on only 8 February. For the "general population limit" dosage the most southerly dispersion on 8 February is 160 km, again well short of US troops.

Turning to potential exposure from fallout due to demolition activity in the Kuwait Theater of Operations we now know that on 4 March 1991 US troops destroyed nerve agent-filled 122mm rockets in Bunker 73 at Khamisiyah. On about 10 March 1991 they also destroyed CW rockets at a Pit area near Khamisiyah. The munitions were not marked at either location and, no acute injuries were reported at the time.

UNSCOM inspected chemical munitions at or near Khamisiyah in October 1991 and identified 122mm sarin/cyclo-sarin (GB/GF) nerve agent-filled rockets and 155mm mustard rounds. At the time, it was not clear whether the chemical weapons identified had been present during the war or whether, as was suspected at other locations, the Iraqis had moved the munitions after the war and just prior to an UNSCOM inspection. The following information was obtained by UNSCOM during its October 1991 inspection.

- At a pit area about 1 km south of the Khamisiyah Storage Area, UNSCOM found several hundred mostly intact 122mm rockets containing nerve agent—detected by sampling and with chemical agent monitors (CAMs).

- In an open area 5 km west of Khamisiyah, inspectors found approximately 6,000 intact 155mm rounds containing mustard agent, as indicated by CAMS.
- At a third location, a single bunker among 100 bunkers, called "Bunker 73" by Iraq, remnants of 122mm rockets were identified.

The Iraqis claimed during the October 1991 inspection that Coalition troops had destroyed Bunker 73 earlier that year. We viewed the Iraqi statements with skepticism at the time because of Baghdad's widespread use of deception against UNSCOM, because we then had so little other intelligence to confirm the Iraqi assertion, and because UNSCOM itself could not verify that chemical weapons had been destroyed until 1996.

CIA concluded in September 1995—after narrowing down to three the number of CW facilities where release might have occurred—identified Khamisiyah as the most probable because of its closer proximity to US forces. We asked the DoD's Investigative Team to look into whether US troops were there. We researched the issue together, and by early March 1996 CIA and DoD developed information that enabled us to believe that US troops did blow up Bunker 73.

The potential exposure of US troops was confirmed on 10 March. On that day, a CIA analyst at home heard a tape recording of a radio show in which a veteran of the 37th Engineering Battalion described demolition activities at a facility that the analyst immediately recognized as Khamisiyah. On 1 May, we briefed the Presidential Advisory Committee that US troops probably destroyed chemical weapons in Bunker 73.

Any remaining doubts that the weapons were chemical were removed by an UNSCOM inspection in May. The UNSCOM inspectors documented the presence of high density polyethylene inserts, burster tubes, fill plugs, and other features characteristic of Iraqi chemical munitions. In addition, during this inspection Iraq told the UNSCOM inspectors that Iraq moved 2,160 *unmarked* 122mm nerve agent rockets to Bunker 73 from the Al Muthanna CW Production and Storage Facility just before the start of the air war. According to Iraq, during the air war they moved about 1,100 rockets from the bunker to the pit area 2 km away. It is important to note that for the first time we were able to corroborate these claims through other sources. We published this information, as well as the results of the modeling of the downwind hazard. These results, as well as the results of the modeling at Muhammadiyat and Al Muthanna, are available on the Internet.

Modeling of the potential hazard caused by destruction of Bunker 73 indicates that an area around the bunker at least 2 km in all directions and 4 km downwind could have been contaminated at or above the level for causing acute symptoms including runny nose, headache, and miosis—that is, constriction of the pupil. An area up to 25 km downwind could have been contaminated at a much lower level. Based on wind models and observations of a video and photographs of destruction activity at Khamisiyah, we determined that the downwind direction was northeast to east.

Some of the modeling assumptions we used were based on data from US testing in 1966. That testing involved destruction of several bunkers filled with GB rockets of similar maximum range to Iraqi rockets found in Bunker 73.

Iraq told UNSCOM in May 1996 that it believed occupying Coalition forces also destroyed some pit area rockets. DoD's investigation into this possibility has showed that US soldiers destroyed stacks of crated munitions in the pit about a week after Bunker 73 was demolished. From analysis of all information, we assess that up to 550 rockets could have been destroyed.

Modeling of the chemical release at the Khamisiyah pit area posed far more difficult challenges than the modeling of other sites. For example, unlike the Bunker 73 demolition, in the pit area we do not know the number or the date of the demolition events, how many shells were destroyed, the wind direction, and other factors critical in determining the dispersion of chemical agents. Moreover, our understanding of several of the important inputs changed while the pit area was being modeled. I would briefly like to go through each one of the areas of uncertainty:

First and most significant, the exact date and numbers of events are still in doubt. We believe that the demolition occurred on 10 March, and there may have been an additional demolition on 12 March. In addition, we know that there were 13 stacks of rockets at the pit area before the destruction activity occurred. However, according to DoD investigators, the number of stacks the soldiers claimed to have destroyed varies from 3 to 9.

- Second, unlike the 4 March event where we had a video, we have no verifiable ground truth showing the wind patterns for 10 or 12 March.

- Third, we have no US testing to indicate the percent of agent released and rate of release for rockets destroyed in the open. For the Bunker 73 demolition, we were able to use the results of earlier US tests of the destruction of artillery rockets in bunkers in our modeling efforts.

- Fourth, in the case of the pit area, a larger amount of agent was released into the atmosphere and evaporation was slower. This further complicated the modeling because weather conditions varied over a longer dispersion period.
- Finally, the pit event is of particular concern because the risk of exposure to US troops was more probable. In the other three releases, the remote location of the event or the northerly direction of the wind are the reasons we believe US troops were not exposed.

As mentioned earlier, we have done about all we can to reduce the uncertainties of the number of munitions destroyed at the pit area. We are now supporting DoD in its effort to model the effects of the demolition activity.

Closing

Let me close by saying that, at this point, analysis by CIA and the Intelligence Community does not support the view that there were other incidents like Khamisiyah. Of course, we will continue to assess any new reports related to possible release of chemical or biological agent in the region.

We will also declassify and make available to the public any new information wherever possible as part of our declassification program. And, more broadly speaking, we are working to increase our resources and expertise on chemical and biological weapons issues. We want to be well-positioned to deal with future contingencies.

The CIA and the DoD teams continue to work together on any chemical and biological warfare aspects of Gulf War illnesses. We inform the Investigative Team of information that might be relevant to chemical or biological exposures. It, in turn, shares its findings with us. If we find information pointing to chemical or biological agent exposures or affecting the issue of Gulf War veterans' illnesses, we will collaborate with DoD to assess those findings.

In closing, I pledge that we will commit whatever intelligence resources are required to support the President and the DoD in their continuing effort to identify the causes of Gulf War Illnesses.

PREPARED STATEMENT OF JOYCE C. LASHOF, M.D., PRESIDENTIAL ADVISORY COMMITTEE ON GULF WAR VETERANS' ILLNESSES

Mr. Chairman, members of the Veterans Affairs Committee, thank you for this opportunity to appear before you today. President Clinton established the Presidential Advisory Committee on Gulf War

41-207 97 - 4

Veterans' Illnesses in May 1995 to ensure an independent, open, and comprehensive examination of health concerns related to Gulf War service. As you know, our *Final Report* to the President was released earlier this week.

The Advisory Committee is a 12-member panel made up of veterans, scientists, health care professionals, and policy experts. We held 18 public meetings between August 1995 and November 1996 and heard invited testimony and received public comment at each meeting. We analyzed information on the full range of activities specified in our charter—research, coordinating efforts, medical treatment, outreach, and risk factors, including chemical and biological weapons. Today I will summarize the Committee's conclusions in three major parts:

- First, an evaluation of the government's response to Gulf War veterans' illnesses;
- Next, an evaluation of available data on the nature of Gulf War veterans' illnesses; and
- Finally, an evaluation of available data on the health effects of Gulf War risk factors.

Because the Committee saw so many parallels with the health concerns of Vietnam veterans, I also will summarize our recommendations on how to avoid similar types of post-conflict health concerns in the future. First, I will provide a summary of our evaluation of the government's response.

Overall, the Committee is encouraged by the government's response to the range of health-related problems experienced by Gulf War veterans. Regarding outreach, we found the Vet Centers and Persian Gulf Family Support Program established by the Department of Veterans Affairs (VA) to be effective outreach programs. We recommend that these field-based initiatives serve as models for health education and risk communication campaigns.

Regarding the clinical evaluation programs, we found them excellent for the diagnosis of Gulf War veterans' illnesses but also found some shortcomings in the availability of treatment. We recommend better follow-up care in the areas of mental health and reproductive health.

Regarding research, the Committee found appropriate emphasis on the epidemiologic studies and studies on stress-related disorders that are most likely to improve our understanding of Gulf War veterans' illnesses. To close gaps in the current knowledge base, we recommend additional research on the long-term health effects of low-level exposures to chemical warfare agents and on the synergistic effects of pyridostigmine bromide. We also recommend more emphasis on basic and applied research on the body's physical response to stress.

I will now provide a summary of our evaluation of the nature and cause of gulf war veterans' illnesses.

Though all the data are not yet in, the Committee was able to reach some conclusions about the nature and cause of Gulf War veterans' illnesses. The Committee made three major findings.

- First, many veterans have illnesses likely to be connected to their service in the Gulf.
- Next, current scientific evidence does not support a causal link between the symptoms and illnesses reported today by Gulf War veterans and exposures while in the Gulf region to the environmental risk factors assessed by the Committee.
- Finally, stress, which is known to affect the brain, immune system, cardiovascular system, and various hormonal responses, is likely to be an important contributing factor to the broad range of physical and psychological illnesses currently being reported by Gulf War veterans.

The Committee looks forward to the results from the large, population-based epidemiologic studies now underway, which will shed additional light on these issues. The Committee also recommends that mortality studies of Gulf War veterans continue, since some health effects, such as cancer, would not be expected to appear until a decade or more after the end of the Gulf War.

Before moving on to recommendations for the future, I have one caveat. I want to emphasize that the Committee takes issue with the government's performance in a key area: investigation of possible exposures of U.S. troops to chemical and biological warfare agents in the Gulf We found substantial evidence of site-specific, low-level exposures to chemical warfare agents. Moreover, we found DOD's investigations to date superficial and unlikely to provide credible answers to veterans' and the public's questions.

As you know, DOD has announced plans to revamp its investigatory and research programs related to low-level chemical warfare agent exposure. We intend to continue our oversight and investigation of these activities with the same vigor that we brought to bear on our evaluation of DOD's prior efforts, generally, as well as on events surrounding Khamisiyah, specifically.

I will now summarize our assessment of the actions needed for the future. The Committee believes the government can do a better job of avoiding post-conflict health concerns. We believe the expertise needed to improve technical performance and implement change resides within the government. But we also believe that DOD and VA have much to learn from their peers in other agencies. Therefore, the Committee recommends that:

- A Presidential Review Directive be issued to instruct the National Science and Technology Council to develop an interagency plan to address health preparedness for and readjustment of veterans and families after future conflicts and peacekeeping missions

This plan needs to have extensive external review. It should address the need for better communication, data, and services, and I would like to highlight a few of the Committee's recommendations in each of these areas.

First, the government clearly needs to work on *better communication* with our service men and women. The volunteers who serve in defense of our Nation deserve complete and accurate information about the risks they face. An open democracy demands that the public, as well, has the opportunity to engage in policy debates that accompany the commitment of troops abroad. Therefore, the Committee recommends that the government:

- develop and implement a comprehensive risk communication plan, and
- solicit timely public and expert comment on any rule that permits waiver of informed consent for use of investigational products in military exigencies.

The government also needs to collect *better data*. Many of the health concerns of Gulf War veterans may never be resolved fully because of the lack of data. To help prevent similar problems in the future, we recommend that officials at the highest echelons assign a high priority to dealing with the problem of lost or missing medical records. We believe the government should develop a protocol for a thorough health evaluation of a large sample of troops to enable better post deployment medical epidemiology. We believe research on possible causes and methods of prevention of excess mortality from external causes among veterans deserves increased attention. And finally, we recommend obtaining data via routine surveys of the reproductive health of military populations.

In the area of *better services*, we believe the government needs to focus its attention to two particular areas. Unfortunately, the government continues to give short shrift to veterans' legitimate concerns about reproductive health. And society at large continues to stigmatize mental health concerns. Therefore, the Committee recommended that the government seek statutory authority to treat veterans and their families for service-connected reproductive problems. And, we recommend that the government continue and intensify efforts to develop stress reduction programs for all troops, with special emphasis on deployed troops.

In conclusion Mr. Chairman and members of the Veterans Affairs Committee, a continued and sustained commitment to a healthy future for Gulf War veterans-for all current and future veterans-is a priority for all Americans. In many important ways the Nation has begun to pay its debt to Gulf War veterans. It is essential, now, to move swiftly toward resolving their principal remaining concerns: How many U.S. troops were exposed to chemical warfare agents, and to what degree?

Thank you again for the opportunity to review our work with you, and I would be happy to answer any questions.

STATEMENT SUBMITTED FOR THE RECORD BY MATTHEW L. PUGLISI, ASSISTANT DIRECTOR FOR GULF WAR VETERANS, VETERANS AFFAIRS AND REHABILITATION COMMISSION, THE AMERICAN LEGION

Mr. Chairman and distinguished members of the Committee:

The American Legion congratulates you on your chairmanship of the Senate Committee on Veterans' Affairs and we also would like to commend you on convening today's hearing investigating Gulf War veterans' illnesses. The Legion is the nation's largest veterans service organization with over 3 million members, and 45,000 of our members are Gulf War veterans. The positive role that your Committee can play cannot be overstated, and we look forward to future hearings in the 105th Congress.

The Gulf War was won after an air war that lasted weeks, and a ground war that only lasted days. For thousands of sick Gulf War veterans and their families, however, the war rages on. Mr. Chairman, in 1991 The American Legion testified before this very Committee concerning the readjustment problems faced by returning Gulf War veterans. We soon learned that the problems confronted by Gulf War veterans were not merely those of readjustment, but health problems as well. It soon became clear to the Legion that many Gulf War veterans began to suffer from poor health as a result of their service in the Persian Gulf. "Many" soon became thousands. The federal government was faced with an overwhelming situation that it met with a mixture of energy in some quarters, and denial in others. Its overall performance was lacking in compassion, and innovative thinking.

Mr. Chairman, congressional oversight has played a major role in improving the federal government's response to Gulf War Illnesses. Now, Congress must ensure that the Department of Veterans Affairs

(VA) and the Department of Defense (DoD) provide quality health care for sick veterans, and aggressively investigate all of the possible risk factors encountered in the Persian Gulf that may have caused these illnesses.

The federal government currently recognizes that tens of thousands of Gulf War veterans are suffering from poor health. Its response has grown exponentially over the last several years. To date, over 80,000 Gulf War veterans have been examined as part of VA's Persian Gulf Health Registry and DoD's Comprehensive Clinical Evaluation Program. VA and DoD also provide health care for symptomatic Gulf War veterans. Over 70 federally funded scientific and clinical studies are underway, or will begin this year, to further examine many of the risk factors present in the Persian Gulf. These efforts, which were mandated by Congress, require Congressional oversight in order to become more effective.

There are several specific programs of VA and DoD, two of the lead agencies of the federal government on Gulf War veterans' illnesses, that need to be investigated by Congress. The Department of Health and Human Services is the third lead agency involved in the issue, and its programs should be overseen as well. This investigation should be conducted with the goal of improving these programs.

VA and DoD Health Care for Sick Gulf War Veterans

How effective is the health care being offered to sick Gulf War veterans? Do Gulf War veterans feel better after they seek care from VA and DoD? Many sick Gulf War veterans who seek care from the government do not receive a diagnosis. This begs the question: how does one successfully treat patients who have undiagnosed illnesses? Neither agency, however, has formally measured outcomes in symptomatic Gulf War veterans who have sought care from the government. The agencies should measure these outcomes, and compare them to outcomes for patients with undiagnosed symptoms in the private sector.

The comparison is important: not only should VA and DoD measure the effectiveness of their health care, they should compare it to the effectiveness of health care provided in the private sector. Treatment methods may exist that VA and DoD are unaware of or have elected to ignore. These treatment methods may ease Gulf War veterans' symptoms while the scientific studies are underway.

Eligibility to Health Care

Until scientific studies determine the cause (or causes) of Gulf War Illnesses, symptomatic Gulf War veterans must remain eligible to receive free health care from VA. Veterans who suffer from these undiagnosed illnesses are not always covered by private health insurance because these illnesses are considered service connected disabilities or pre-existing conditions. In order to ensure these sick veterans have access to care, Congress should allow VA to care for these veterans who are disabled from their service.

The American Legion recognizes that some family members of sick Gulf War veterans have developed illnesses similar to the sick veteran in their family. The Legion is also concerned by adverse birth outcomes in female Gulf War veterans and spouses of male Gulf War veterans, to include miscarriages and birth defects. Their poor health and birth defects may stem directly from the veteran's service in the Gulf and, therefore, they should be entitled to VA or DoD health care at no cost to the veteran, until an association can be established.

Compensation: Persian Gulf Undiagnosed Illness Claims

Three reports, including one prepared by The American Legion, found flaws in the adjudication of VA disability compensation claims for Gulf War veterans who did not receive a diagnosis from a VA medical doctor. VA has recently reopened all of these claims, and is seeking additional evidence and supporting documentation from these veterans so it can reconsider the claims. The American Legion commends VA on this effort to correct these problems in such a sweeping and aggressive manner. This Committee *must* conduct oversight hearings to assess the success of this review.

The American Legion applauds the President's recent announcement that he has directed the Secretary of Veterans Affairs to evaluate increasing the two year presumptive period for Gulf War undiagnosed illness claims. The American Legion adamantly opposed the two year presumptive period when Public Law 103–446 was debated in the 103rd Congress. That law allowed VA to pay disability compensation to Gulf War veterans suffering from undiagnosed illnesses, and whose symptoms became manifest within two years of their departure from the Gulf. It was clear to us then, as it is now, that the government should not limit the presumptive period before the science determines what Gulf War veterans are suffering from. The two year period was arrived at arbitrarily and must be expanded. A longer period gives the benefit of the doubt to the veterans, who suffer from something that may manifest itself outside the two year presumptive period. This proposal would not open the treasury to undeserving veterans, as some may argue. It would allow service connected disabled veterans to receive the compensation to which they are entitled.

Risk Factors

There are a number of risk factors encountered by troops in the Persian Gulf that have been identified as possible causes for Gulf War Illnesses. They include:

- chemical warfare agents
- biological warfare agents
- stress
- pyridostigmine bromide
- smoke from oil well fires
- vaccines
- indigenous infectious disease
- depleted uranium
- pesticides
- petroleum products

The American Legion recognizes that sick Gulf War veterans were stationed all over the theater of operations. Some were exposed to all or few of the risk factors, and yet all report poor health. It is unjustified to favor one risk factor above any of the others until the scientific studies are completed. Some appear more likely than the others, especially for veterans who experienced particular exposures. Judgment and speculation are best reserved at the end of the investigative process, not the beginning.

Yesterday's announcement by Dr. Robert Haley, of the University of Texas, is an example of why rushing to judgment does a disservice to veterans and science. Dr. Haley found objective signs of nerve damage in symptomatic Gulf War veterans who reported exposure to pyridostigmine bromide, pesticides, and chemical warfare agents. The lesson from Dr. Haley's findings is that the principal risk factor favored by the Presidential Advisory Committee, stress, was found not to be a plausible risk factor by Dr. Haley.

The American Legion is disturbed by reports that medical doctors employed by VA, who have proposed "unorthodox" theories concerning Gulf War Illnesses, are being pressured by VA to "toe the line." We are equally concerned with the media's narrow focus on the issue to the exclusion of reporting on the important issues confronting sick Gulf War veterans, like access to health care and disability compensation. Suppressing open discussion, debate, and research into plausible theories will prevent the scientific community, in the long run, from understanding why Gulf War veterans are sick. Focusing on just one risk factor, to the exclusion of others, will do the same. The Committee should ensure that it remains open to all the risk factors, and plausible theories, and it should encourage all of the federal agencies involved to do the same.

Stress as a Risk Factor

Stress has been offered as a likely risk factor that may have caused illness in the majority of symptomatic veterans by the Presidential Advisory Committee and by Dr. Kenneth Hyams (*Annals of Internal Medicine,* Sept. 1996) to name a few. Some observers have claimed that Gulf War veterans reject stress as playing *any* role in the illnesses. Gulf War Illnesses were initially *dismissed* as stress-related by government medical doctors on too many occasions immediately following the war. Veterans' anger concerning stress is not directed at the role it may play in their poor health, but how their poor health was dismissed as stress-related early on.

The American Legion played a major role in the effort to recognize Post Traumatic Stress Disorder (PTSD) as a real disease that affects thousands who serve in combat. PTSD is a well defined psychological illness that affects some who encounter traumatic events. It is found not only in combat veterans, but in police officers, firefighters, rape victims, and abused children. There are well known and effective treatments for PTSD, and these treatments are most effective if they are sought during the early stages of the illness. The American Legion continues to reach out to those veterans who suffer from it and we encourage them to seek treatment for an illness that has occurred since wars have been fought. We will continued to do our utmost to remove the stigma attached to any psychological illness suffered by veterans, particularly PTSD. PTSD afflicts warriors, not weaklings, and through our efforts, thousands of veterans who initially rejected the PTSD diagnosis are receiving treatment at VA and leading more productive lives.

We therefore take exception to charges by some observers that veterans are rejecting stress as a likely cause of Gulf War Illnesses because they want to "legitimize" Gulf War Illnesses by blaming them on chemical exposures. If we advised veterans who are diagnosed with and actually suffer from PTSD to rule out stress as a legitimate risk factor, we wouldn't be true veterans' advocates

Thousands of Gulf War veterans suffer from PTSD. Many have been identified and are receiving treatment from VA or private doctors. But PTSD does *not* explain the range of illnesses observed in symptomatic Gulf War veterans who do not have a diagnosis. If they had PTSD, their symptoms would not go undiagnosed.

Recent studies and ongoing ones have found that stress may affect the human body's biochemistry. This, in turn, may cause certain drugs (pyridostigmine bromide), toxins (sarin) or the combination to behave differently in the body than scientists have observed in the quiet setting of a laboratory. This has been shown to be the case in rodents in a recently published Israeli study.

Stress has also been shown to weaken the human immune system. The theory as applied to Gulf War veterans is that the stress of service in the Gulf may have permitted opportunistic infections to occur in Gulf War veterans; infections that may continue to disable. Chemicals and drugs encountered in the Gulf may have behaved differently because troops in the Gulf were under stress.

Gulf War veterans recognize that stress *may* play a role in causing some of these physiological illnesses, although what role, if any, should be determined by the ongoing scientific studies. The Committee is encouraged to investigate the role of stress, but like any other risk factor, it should not do so to the exclusion of the others.

The findings of Dr. Haley strengthen this position of the veterans. Dr. Haley's rigorous scientific methods leave little room for doubt in the veterans he studied: stress did not play a role in their disease. He found *none* who suffered from PTSD.

DoD's Use of Investigational Drugs

With some studies suggesting pyridostigmine bromide's (PB) role in Gulf War veterans' illnesses, and many more underway that are investigating PB's role, DoD should immediately end the use of PB as a nerve agent prophylactic. The American Legion would also like to urge Congress to conduct oversight of DoD's efforts to implement procedures regarding the distribution, record keeping and tracking of inoculations and investigational drugs for future conflicts.

Depleted Uranium

Thousands of Depleted Uranium (DU) munitions were fired or set on fire in the Persian Gulf. DU is a radioactive and chemically toxic material. Thousands of Gulf War veterans may have been exposed to DU particles before, during and after the war. Although its relation to the current illnesses is unknown, DoD has not properly investigated whether or not DU could cause short or long term illness of veterans exposed to it. Given the proliferation of DU throughout the world and DoD's reliance on it for future conflicts, this investigation must begin immediately. Gulf War veterans will not be the last Americans exposed to DU on the battlefield and we should not remain ignorant of its possible health affects any longer.

Presidential Advisory Committee on Gulf War Veterans' Illnesses Final Report

The American Legion would urge the Committee to thoughtfully review the Presidential Advisory Committee on Gulf War Veterans' Illnesses (PAC) Final Report and ensure that all of its recommendations are implemented by the federal government. The American Legion believes that the PAC was instrumental in forcing

DoD to reconsider its position on various issues, especially with regards to chemical and biological warfare agent exposures.

The President's extension of the PAC will ensure another oversight tool is in place, one that has been successful to date. The American Legion welcomes this extension and encourages the Committee and Congress to work closely with the PAC in the months ahead.

Tissue/Serum Sampling and CBW Exposures

Reports from the United Nations and the Pentagon state that U.S. troops in the Gulf were possibly exposed to chemical warfare agents. As a result of a recent U.N. report concerning Iraq's biological warfare program and Iraqi weaponization of aflatoxin, a biological warfare agent, the Pentagon now admits that it does not know for certain whether service personnel were exposed to biological warfare agents. In light of these new revelations, The American Legion believes that tissue from Gulf War veterans should be collected and stored until biological markers can be identified to determine whether sick veterans were exposed to chemical and biological warfare agents. Studies will soon be underway to determine whether exposure to low levels of nerve and mustard agents can cause long term illness. The missing piece of the puzzle is exposure data which would help researchers determine dose levels. In other words, no one knows how much of these agents U.S. troops were exposed to in the Gulf, or in the case of aflatoxin, whether they were exposed at all. Tissue sampling, if conducted soon and in a thoughtful manner, could help answer this question.

Tissue samples were not collected from Vietnam veterans exposed to Agent Orange until a biological marker for dioxin was isolated in 1988. By then, it was too late to determine dose levels in Vietnam veterans because it had been so long since their exposure. Had tissue been collected and frozen immediately following the war, these samples could have been thawed in 1988 and analyzed. Medical doctors and Vietnam veterans could have learned the level of their exposure to dioxin during the war. Vietnam veterans, however, will probably never know. The American Legion and Vietnam veterans have learned a hard lesson from the Agent Orange tragedy on the issue of tissue samples. Biological markers for chemical and biological agents encountered in the Persian Gulf may be isolated soon, or not perhaps for many years; however, we *must* collect tissue samples today.

Investigation of Exposures to Chemical and Biological Weapons

The American Legion believes DoD should not investigate itself concerning the issue of chemical and biological warfare agent exposures and incidences during the Persian Gulf War without credible oversight. Missing logs; slow release of information; and repeated denials for several years in the face of overwhelming evidence all have combined to undermine the credibility of DoD. DoD's current efforts and devotion of resources are impressive and appear sincere. Dr. Bernard Rostker and his team must be commended on their early efforts to communicate with the veterans community and listen to our concerns. However, The American Legion would like to remind this Committee that these current efforts, like past DoD efforts, are the result of immense pressure from Congress, the PAC, The American Legion and sick Gulf War veterans. DoD views the Khamisiyah announcement as a "watershed event" and it appears to be pursuing the President's call to "leave no stone unturned." It would be of great benefit to DoD and the federal government as a whole, if a congressionally appointed independent commission, with subpoena powers, oversees this investigation.

In 1994, DoD, VA and HHS assured veterans that no classified documents existed that pointed to possible exposures to chemical and biological weapons. That assurance turned out to be false. Worse, classified logs maintained at Central Command are missing and these missing logs cover periods during which key events occurred. The same is true of tapes from FOX vehicles that recorded chemical warfare agent detections. Any investigation must explain why DoD's earlier investigations were such absolute failures and why classified logs are missing. The entire Department is not at fault, but only certain individuals who apparently misinformed three members of the Cabinet. They should be identified and questioned about their actions or lack thereof. The American Legion notes that individuals who lose or misplace classified materials, such as combat logs, have violated the Uniform Code of Military Justice and other federal laws.

Too much is at stake. The shine of the great victory in the Gulf has been tarnished by bureaucratic bumbling, at best or a deliberate effort to conceal the truth, at worst. Only independent investigators with subpoena powers and without a vested interest can vouch for the accuracy of any final report from DoD. We all want to see DoD succeed in restoring its credibility. This is how it can best be done.

U.S. Preparedness to Fight a Chemical and Biological War

The evidence from before, during and after the Gulf War suggest that the U.S. military is woefully unprepared to fight an adversary armed with such weapons. The Department of Defense *must* devote more planning and resources into developing strategies and equipment that alert and protect our troops against these weapons of mass destruction. More importantly, DoD should consider changes in the military's warfighting doctrine regarding the detection of and protection from sub-acute levels of chemical and biological warfare agents. The American Legion believes the inadequacy of U.S. forces to effectively detect chemical and biological warfare agents and protect military personnel from low level chemical and biological warfare agent exposures represents a serious national security issue which must be addressed.

Mr. Chairman, legislation, appropriations and federal regulations allow the federal government to care and compensate Gulf War veterans and require it to seek the cause for their illnesses. However, oversight is the tool to ensure VA and DoD fulfill these mandates and resolve these issues. Mr. Chairman, The American Legion and sick Gulf War veterans and their families truly appreciate your leadership on this issue. This concludes my testimony.

STATEMENT SUBMITTED FOR THE RECORD BY DENNIS CULLINAN, DEPUTY DIRECTOR, NATIONAL LEGISLATIVE SERVICE, VETERANS OF FOREIGN WARS OF THE UNITED STATES

Mr. Chairman and members of the Committee:

On behalf of the 2.1 million men and women of the Veterans of Foreign Wars, I thank you for the opportunity to express the views of the VFW on the very important matter of illnesses that are affecting a number of our Persian Gulf veterans. The VFW has worked diligently in the effort to resolve this controversial issue, and will continue to do so until a resolution is reached that appropriately cares for the veterans involved. I would also like to take this time to extend to you, Mr. Chairman, the VFW's congratulations on your appointment as the Chairman of the Senate Veterans Affairs Committee. We look forward to working with you on all veterans matters and know you will do whatever is necessary to ensure that the nation's veterans are cared for appropriately.

Mr. Chairman, the VFW wholeheartedly agrees with you that the current two-year presumptive period for undiagnosed illnesses associated with service in the Gulf is, at this time, unwarranted. After consultation with VA as to the reasons for the two-year presumptive period, the VFW, on October 3, 1996, sent a communiqué to Secretary of VA Jesse Brown calling instead for the establishment of an open-ended presumptive period. The VFW believes that in light of current medical and scientific data, or, more appropriately, lack thereof, in conjunction with the experiences reported by Gulf War veterans themselves, it is far too early to establish a time limit as to when exposure symptoms will manifest.

We are pleased that Secretary Brown has agreed to our request, and the request of the Committee. We do urge, however, that such a change be implemented at the earliest possible date. If Secretary Brown is unable to do so—he spoke of a 60 day review period to determine the appropriate length of the presumptive period—then possibly this is something that should be done legislatively. (It is our understanding, however, that Secretary Brown does have the authority to implement such a change per Public Law 103–446.) The VFW will, nonetheless, most assuredly assist the Committee in ensuring that the necessary changes are made at the earliest possible date.

On a related matter, the VFW is extremely concerned about the denial rate for veterans seeking service-connection for "undiagnosed illnesses" as a result of service in the Gulf Out of the over 10,000 Gulf War veterans who have been rated for an "undiagnosed illness" claim (Gulf War Illness), only 529 have been service-connected for compensation. (It is likely that the restrictive presumptive period concerning the manifestation of the condition is the primary reason why 95% of all "Undiagnosed-Illness" claims have been denied.)

Given the number of Gulf War veterans who have come forward with claims of illnesses that have yet to be diagnosed, it seems implausible to us that 95% of them have no basis for an "undiagnosed illness" service-connected rating. And while it is our understanding that a number of these veterans are in fact service-connected for other diagnosable ailments attributable to their service in the Gulf, we have great concern for those who are left out in the cold. And as for those who are service-connected for other diagnosable illnesses, there is the risk that they may be not receiving the appropriate treatment for any undiagnosable ailment not deemed service-connected.

The VFW has brought up this matter with VA and the Presidential Advisory Committee on Gulf War Veterans' Illnesses (PACGWVI). In an effort to ensure that no Persian Gulf veteran suffering from any degree of an undiagnosable illness goes uncompensated, we have promoted the need for some type of case definition for "Gulf War Syndrome." Unfortunately, this proposal has been met mostly with resistance. And while we are aware of the intricate problems associated with such an undertaking, we feel the alternatives situation where individual Persian Gulf veterans might go uncompensated for an undiagnosed illness associated with their service in the Gulf is far more unacceptable.

Mr. Chairman, the VFW has also pushed for the extension of the President's Advisory Committee on Gulf War Veterans' Illnesses beyond its original date of termination, scheduled for the end of 1996. We are very pleased that the President has recognized the excellent work done by the Advisory Committee and has granted our request, extending the life of the Advisory Committee for another nine months. Furthermore, we also pushed hard for the President to extend to the Advisory Committee additional oversight powers, another request which he granted. Given that certain governmental entities have been less than forthcoming with relevant data and slothful in enacting the appropriate measures, we felt this was a necessary act.

Lastly, the VFW supports you and the other members of the Veterans Affairs Committee with regard to the role of stress in the undiagnosed illnesses. While it may be true that stress does play a part in these ailments, we find it unfathomable as well as counterproductive to insist that stress is the predominant cause. To say that these ailments are nothing more than in the veterans' heads is an insult. We hope that as the medical and scientific community hones in on the causes and remedies of these illnesses, that they are not restricted by the notion that stress is the cause. It would only result in an extreme and potentially dangerous disservice to our ill veterans.

Mr. Chairman, the VFW is pleased that the appropriate amount of attention is being paid to resolving this issue. We feel that with the support of persons such as yourself and the rest of the Senate Veterans Affairs Committee, we can find a solution that adequately cares for those veterans whose current ill situation resulted from their unselfish acts for the good of our nation. Again, on behalf of the Veterans of Foreign Wars of the United States, I thank you for the opportunity to be heard on this most important issue. Thank you.

CORRESPONDENCE SUBMITTED FOR THE RECORD BY THE DISABLED AMERICAN VETERANS

Motto: "If I cannot speak good of my comrade, I will not speak ill of him."

DISABLED AMERICAN VETERANS

NATIONAL SERVICE and LEGISLATIVE HEADQUARTERS
807 MAINE AVENUE, S.W.
WASHINGTON, D.C. 20024
(202) 554-3501

January 14, 1997

Honorable Arlen Specter, Chairman
Senate Veterans' Affairs Committee
711 Hart Senate Office Building
Washington, D.C. 20510-6375

Dear Chairman Specter:

I take this opportunity to commend you, Ranking Democratic Member John D. "Jay" Rockefeller, IV, and those members of your committee who participated in the Senate Veterans' Affairs Committee hearing on Thursday, January 9, 1997, concerning Persian Gulf War veterans. It was obvious from the way you conducted this hearing that you have strong feelings and concerns about the health and well-being of Persian Gulf War veterans.

Like you, the Disabled American Veterans is concerned about the health and well-being of Persian Gulf War veterans and their ability to obtain benefits. From the beginning, we have expressed our concerns about a closed presumptive period for undiagnosed illnesses. It has been our firm belief that since no one knows the etiology of the undiagnosed illnesses suffered by Persian Gulf War veterans, that it is unrealistic to state that this disability must manifest within a specific period of years following service in the Persian Gulf.

We wholeheartedly agree that the presumptive period as prescribed under 38 U.S.C. § 1117 must be expanded beyond the current two-year period. We would caution your committee, however, to allow the Secretary of Veterans Affairs to do so on his own. Should Congress pass remedial legislation to expand the current two-year presumptive period for undiagnosed illnesses, there would certainly be "pay-go" implications which would have an adverse impact on other Department of Veterans Affairs' programs.

We look forward to working with you, the other members of the Senate Veterans' Affairs Committee and VA Secretary Jesse Brown to ensure that this matter is expeditiously handled and that no Persian Gulf War veteran is irreparably harmed.

Sincerely,

DAVID W. GORMAN
Executive Director, Washington Headquarters

DWG:lmb

POSTHEARING QUESTIONS FROM CHAIRMAN SPECTER TO THE DEPARTMENT OF VETERANS AFFAIRS AND THE RESPONSES

Question 1. Officials from the VA, the Department of Defense and Health and Human Services were organized into a Persian Gulf Veterans Coordinating Board at the beginning of 1994. Since its inception, how effective do you feel it has been in facilitating the sharing of information between these Departments and avoiding duplication of efforts?

Answer. In January 1994, the President established the Persian Gulf Veterans Coordinating Board, chaired by the Secretaries of the Department of Veterans Affairs (VA), Department of Defense (DoD), and Department of Health and Human Services (HHS), to provide interdepartmental coordination and direction of federal programs related to Persian Gulf War veterans. The Coordinating Board provides an interdepartmental means to share information on Persian Gulf War veterans' health, to allocate available resources to the apparent highest priorities, to avoid duplication of efforts, and to disseminate new research information. The Coordinating Board has been highly effective at accomplishing these four specific objectives:

- to ensure that all veterans are provided the complete range of health care services necessary to take care of medical problems that may be related to deployment in Operations Desert Shield and Desert Storm. Providing appropriate medical care has been a top priority of VA and DoD. The two departments have acted aggressively to ensure the delivery of high quality medical care to Persian Gulf veterans.

- to develop a research program that will result in the most accurate and complete understanding of the health problems experienced by Persian Gulf War veterans and the factors that have contributed to these problems. There are currently 90 government research projects, in various stages of progress, focusing on the highest priority medical and scientific issues. More than 30 of these projects are VA-sponsored.

- to develop clear and consistent guidelines for the evaluation and compensation of disabilities related to Persian Gulf service. VA and DoD continue to work diligently to ensure prompt and appropriate compensation to Persian Gulf veterans disabled by their military service.

- to ensure that Persian Gulf veterans and their health care providers have access to the latest information on medical care, compensation, and research. This information enables veterans to make sound judgments about their own health status, and to know how and where they can seek assistance. It also enables physicians and other health care providers to provide accurate diagnoses and effective treatment to veterans.

VA plays a central role in the Persian Gulf Veterans Coordinating Board through its participation in the Clinical, Research, and Compensation and Benefits Working Groups. In particular, the Research Working Group provides guidance and coordination for VA, DoD and HHS research activities related to Persian Gulf War veterans' health. It coordinates all research studies conducted or sponsored by these three departments to prevent unnecessary duplication and to ensure that important gaps in scientific knowledge are identified and addressed. The working group is actively involved in directing resources toward high priority questions and monitoring the results of federally-sponsored research projects. It has, in our opinion, been very effective in this role. It has produced two reports: the *Report of Federal Research_Activities Related to Persian Gulf Veterans Illnesses* and the 1996 update of *A Working Plan for Research On Persian Gulf Veterans Illnesses.*

The Persian Gulf Veterans Coordinating Board has been a valuable interagency activity. It has served its coordination mission very well in health care, research and compensation of Gulf War veterans.

Question 2. Secretary Brown's testimony referred to a group of on-site Khamisiyah demolition teams numbering 81 persons with musculoskeletal conditions at a higher rate than the general registry group. Please specify for the Committee the nature of these conditions, how much higher a rate it was and, if you would, comment on the possible significance of these findings.

Answer. With regard to the probable troop exposure to chemical warfare nerve agents, the Department of Defense provided VA with a list of 21,799 individuals who they identified likely being present within 50 kilometers of the Khamisiyah Ammunition Storage Area during the demolition period in March 1991. A computer match of the Persian Gulf Health Examination Registry database with this list identified 1,978 veterans, or approximately 9 percent, who had completed Registry examinations prior to September 1996. A comparison of the examination results of these individuals with other Registry participants shows that similar types and rates of symptoms, diagnoses, and self-reported health status are reported, but virtually no individual in this group reported no symptoms at the time of their Registry examinations. Furthermore, the eighty-one Registry participants who are identified as part of the on-site Khamisiyah demolition team, report symptoms classified as musculoskeletal conditions (muscle pain, joint pain), at a higher rate than the 50 kilometer or general Registry groups. A comparison of the three groups is shown below.

Complaint	*All Registry Exams**	*50km (N=1,978) %*	*On-Site (N=81) %*
Muscle, Joint Pain	16.8%	18.4%	28.4%

* "All Registry Exams" data as of January 1996; 50 km and on-site data include examinations through September 1996. (Data prepared by VA Environmental Epidemiology Service)

Attached is a table outlining the specific diagnoses listed in the Registry database for the eighty-one members of the Khamisiyah demolition team.

ATTACHMENT

List of Diseases Diagnosed by Examining Physicians Among
24 Veterans Complaining of Muscle and Joint Pain

Personal I.D.	Diagnoses
6	Other unspecified joint disorder/Disease due to virus
7	Dermatophytosis on foot/Other derangement of joint
8	No Diagnoses
11	Osteoarthrosis
15	Other unspecified joint disorders/Disorders of lipid metabolism/Intestinal disorder
16	No Diagnoses
23	Adjustment disorder/Other unspecified arthropathies
24	Sprained hand/Osteoarthrosis
28	No Diagnoses
30	No Diagnoses
31	Sacroiliitis/Psoriasis/Other disease due to virus
32	No Diagnoses
33	Rheumatoid arthritis/Dermatophytosis on foot/Neurotic depression
34	Reiter's disease (VD)/ Unspecified gastritis
35	No Diagnoses
38	Inguinal hernia
42	Degeneration of lumbar of lumbosacral intervertebral disc/ esophageal reflux
43	Tineanigra
51	Pain in joint (Arthralgia)/ Myalgia and myositis, unspecified
55	Other inflammatory disorders of male genital organs
58	No Diagnoses
62	Lipoma (unspecified site)
63	No Diagnoses
71	Lumbago/Asthma (unspecified)/Internal hemorrhoids without mention of complication

LIST OF DISEASES DIAGNOSED BY EXAMINING PHYSICIANS AMONG 57 VETERANS WITHOUT COMPLAINTS OF MUSCLE AND JOINT PAIN

#1 - Tietze's disease/anxiety state, unspecified/agranulocytosis

#2 - Brachial neuritis or radiculilitis NOS/Urticaria, unspecified

#3 - Other acne (diseases of sebaceous gland)

#4 - Asthma, unspecified/irritable colon

#5 - No diagnosis

#9 - No diagnosis

#10 - Malignant neoplasm of brain stem

#12 - Fracture of unspecified part of femur/disorder of lumbago/unspecified hearing loss

#13 - Pain in joint (arthralgia)

#14 - Trigeminal nerve disorder, unspecified/pure hypercholesterolemia

#17 - Anxiety state, unspecified

#18 - No diagnosis

#19 - Hematuria

#20 - No diagnosis

#21 - No diagnosis

#22 - Alopecia, unspecified

#25 - No diagnosis

#26 - Essential hypertension, benign/unspecified sinusitis (chronic)/unspecified disorder of lipid metabolism

#27 - Pure hypercholesterolemia (of lipoid metabolism)/other diseases of lung, not elsewhere classified (broncholithiasis, calcification of lung, lung disease NOS, pulmolithiasis)

#29 - Essential hypertension, benign/other acne (diseases of sebaceous glands)/contusion of unspecified site

#36 - No diagnosis

#37 - Unspecified local infection of skin and subcutaneous tissue

#39 - Other non-specific abnormal serum enzyme levels/abnormal finds on radiological and other examinations of lung field

#40 - Asthma unspecified

#41 - Unspecified disorder of synovium, tendon, and bursa/unspecified gastritis and gastroduodenitis/diaphragmatic hernia

#44 - Non-specific elevation of levels of transaminase or lactic acid dehydrogenase (LDH)

#45 - No diagnosis

#46 - Alopecia unspecified

#47 - Osteoarthrosis, unspecified whether localized or generalized/fracture of distal end of humerous, other (multiple fractures of lower end, trochlea)

#48 - Other acne (diseases of sebaceous gland)/flat foot/pain in joint (arthralgia)

#49 - Dermatophytosis of foot

#50 - Fracture of unspecified part of neck of femur, open/late effect of internal injury to intra abdominal organs/osteoarthrosis, unspecified whether general or localized

#52 - Depressive disorder, not elsewhere classified/prolonged post traumatic stress disorder

#53	-	Conjunctivitis, unspecified
#54	-	No diagnosis
#56	-	No diagnosis
#57	-	No diagnosis
#59	-	Calculus of kidney/osteoarthrosis, unspecified whether generalized or localized
#60	-	Other forms of migraine
#61	-	Exotropia
#64	-	Other diseases of the lung not elsewhere classified
#65	-	Dyschromia
#66	-	Anal fissure/essential hypertension, unspecified/allergic rhinitis due to pollen
#67	-	Unspecified sinusitis (chronic)/variants of migraine
#68	-	No diagnosis
#69	-	No diagnosis
#70	-	Disorder of lumbago/cervicobrachial syndrome (diffuse)/psychalgia-headache tension
#72	-	No diagnosis
#73	-	No diagnosis
#74	-	Depressive disorder not elsewhere classified
#75	-	Alopecia, unspecified
#76	-	Depressive disorder not elsewhere classified/cardiac dysrhythmia, unspecified

#77 - Hyperplasia of prostate/traumatic arthropathy/prolonged post traumatic stress disorder

#78 - Scar conditions and fibrosis of skin

#79 - No numbers

#80 - Unspecified functional disorder of stomach/unspecified hypothyroidism/hepatitis C

#81 - Unspecified adverse effect of drug, medicinal, and biological substance

This health surveillance data is preliminary and is compiled from evaluations of a non-random, self-selected group of the individuals possibly exposed to nerve agents at Khamisiyah. While this information gives a partial snapshot of the health of some veterans thought to be present at this site in March 1991, the results should not be generalized to the entire Khamisiyah group or considered definitive. VA does not consider these differences as indicative of a causal link between the Gulf War veterans' illnesses and chemical warfare agent exposure, nor do we consider these differences significant at the present time. More complete information on the potential exposures, and the individuals affected, and research on the possible chronic health effects of low-level chemical warfare nerve agent exposures are needed.

POST HEARING QUESTION FROM SENATOR CAMPBELL TO THE DEPARTMENT OF VETERANS AFFAIRS AND THE RESPONSES

Question 1. Mr. Secretary, this question pertains to the benefits and claims of Persian Gulf War Veterans. Since the end of the Persian Gulf War to December 1996, the Western Region of the VA reports the following—

- it has rated 1,813 Persian Gulf War Veterans claims,
- granted 174 claims,
- partially granted 264 claims,
- denied 1,375 claims, and

Colorado's VA has reported the following—

- it has rated 343 Persian Gulf War Veterans claims,
- granted 33 claims,
- partially granted 54 claims,
- denied 256 claims.

(a) If you do the math, the VA is denying Persian Gulf War veterans claims in the Western Region at a rate of 73% and in Colorado specifically at a rate of 74.6%. If these numbers are correct, are they consistent with the national average?

(b) Can you explain this high denial rate Persian Gulf War veterans' claims, especially in light of the fact that they are to receive care even if their illness is still undiagnosed?

(c) If these numbers are not accurate, would you please provide them to the Committee, along with justifications?

Answer. The numbers quoted by Senator Campbell are taken from the tracking system used to monitor Persian Gulf veterans' compensation claims based on exposure to environmental hazards or adjudicated under the regulation specific to undiagnosed illnesses. They reflect the results of claims considered under both sets of criteria. These types of claims are handled in 4 regional offices, one in each of VBA's 4 administrative areas. These regional offices, known as Area Processing Offices (APOs), are Philadelphia (Eastern Area), Louisville (Central Area), Nashville (Southern Area), and Phoenix (Western Area).

The numbers show that of the 1,813 veterans whose claims based on environmental hazards have been adjudicated in the Western Area, 24 percent have established service connection for at least one disability related to either an environmental hazard or an undiagnosed illness. Among Colorado veterans specifically, 25.4 percent have established service connection. Nationally, of the 11,257 veterans' claims considered at the 4 APOs, 1,391 (12.4 percent) have established service connection for at least one disability related to either an environmental hazard or an undiagnosed illness. These numbers indicate that the Western Area and the Denver Regional Office are doing relatively well with this type of claim.

Denial of claims based on undiagnosed illnesses are categorized in our tracking system under one of the following reasons:

- the disability is determined to be the result of a diagnosed condition;
- the evidence indicates that the illness causing the disability is not chronic;
- the disability has been found to be due to a reason unrelated to service in the Persian Gulf;
- the disability did not manifest itself during service in the Persian Gulf or within the current 2-year presumptive period thereafter;
- no disability is shown by the current evidence of record; and
- the evidence indicates that a disability, first appearing within the presumptive period, has never been 10 percent disabling.

However, we do not agree that there is a high denial rate of Persian Gulf veterans' claims. In many instance, disabilities claimed to result from environmental hazards or undiagnosed illnesses form only one part of a veteran's total compensation claim. Recent statistics on all types of compensation claims received from Persian Gulf veterans disclose that 65,000 of 84,147 veterans (77 percent) have been awarded service connection for one or more disabilities. Of these, 27,300 (32 percent) are in receipt of compensation; another 37,700 (45 percent) have a zero percent rating, indicating that a service-connected disability exists although it is not compensable. Of course, Persian Gulf veterans who have zero percent service-connected evaluations may receive medical care for those conditions. All Persian Gulf veterans may receive medical care for conditions that might possibly be the result of exposure to a toxic substance or environmental hazard during their Gulf service. This eligibility of Persian Gulf veterans for medical care is separate from potential entitlement to service connection.

For your additional information, we are in the midst of a readjudication of the 11,000 Persian Gulf undiagnosed illness cases identified in the tracking system. This readjudication was begun in July 1996 and is intended to ensure that all Persian Gulf veterans are aware of and have an opportunity to submit all types of evidence that may establish entitlement to service connection. We have also taken steps to ensure that the information entered into the tracking system is correct and provides an accurate picture of the final outcomes in these claims. We anticipate that the readjudication will be complete by the Fall of this year.

POSTHEARING QUESTIONS FROM SENATOR JEFFORDS TO THE DEPARTMENT OF VETERANS AFFAIRS AND THE RESPONSES

Question 1. Officials from the VA, the Departments of Defense and Health and Human Services were organized into a Persian Gulf Veterans Coordinating Board at the beginning of 1994. Since its inception, how effective do you feel it has been in facilitating the sharing of information between these Departments and avoiding duplication of efforts?

Answer. Since its establishment in January 1994, the Persian Gulf Veterans Coordinating Board has been instrumental in improving the communication and coordination of activities related to Persian Gulf War veterans. The main function of the Coordinating Board is to provide direction and ensure coordination among the Departments of Veterans Affairs, Defense, and Health and Human Services on all issues related to Persian Gulf veterans, health matters. The Coordinating Board serves as a vehicle to break down institutional barriers which hamper communication between these organizations with their differing individual missions. It assures that the independent Departmental efforts are moving forward in a complimentary and effective manner. The Department of Veterans Affairs views the Board as a valuable tool for future interagency veterans, health efforts and supports the concept of enlarging the mission of the Board to encompass deployment planning and medical surveillance for future military missions.

Question 2. Secretary Brown's testimony referred to a group of on-site Khamisiyah demolition teams numbering 81 persons with musculoskeletal conditions at a higher rate than the general registry group. Please specify for the Committee the nature of these conditions, how much higher a rate it was and, if you would, comment on the possible significance of these findings.

Answer. In an attempt to better understand the possible health consequences of service in the vicinity of the Khamisiyah Ammunition Storage Area during the demolition activity which occurred in March 1991, VA did some exploratory analysis of its Persian Gulf Registry Health Examination database. The Department of Defense had provided VA with a list of 21,799 individuals whom they identified as possibly being present within 50 kilometers of Khamisiyah during this period. A computer match of the Registry database with this list identified 1,978 veterans, or approximately 9 percent, that had completed Registry exams prior to September 1996. A comparison of the examination results of these individuals with other Registry participants showed similar types of symptoms, diagnoses, and self-reported health status, but virtually all veterans in the Khamisiyah group were symptomatic. Furthermore, the 81 Registry participants who were identified to us by DoD as being members of the demolition team reported symptoms and were diagnosed with musculoskeletal conditions at a higher rate than the 50 kilometer group or the general Registry participant group. For muscle and joint pain symptoms this represented 28.4 percent, 18.4 percent and 16.8 percent, respectively. The frequency of medical conditions which are classified within the International Classification of Diseases (ICD) diagnostic category of "Musculoskeletal and Connective Tissue Diseases" was 30.9 percent for demolition team members, 25.9 percent for the veterans within 50 kilometers of Khamisiyah, plus 25.9 percent for general Registry participants. A review of VA hospital admissions files (PTF database) did not reveal a similar pattern in increased frequency of hospitalizations for a diagnosis of musculoskeletal conditions in the Khamisiyah demolition team members.

The Registry examinations represent a large clinical case series. The health surveillance data provided by the above analysis is preliminary and compiled from health evaluations on a non-random, self-selected group of individuals possibly exposed to the nerve agents sarin and cyclosarin. While this information gives a limited view of the health of some veterans thought to be present at this site in March 1991, the results should not be generalized to the entire Khamisiyah group nor be considered to be caused by nerve agent exposure. Contrary to certain media reports, this data does not provide evidence of a causal link between the illnesses of Registry veterans and exposure to nerve agents. We do not believe it is possible to establish any type of causation based on the differences identified among these Registry participants. A number of risk factors, other than chemical warfare exposure, may be responsible for the identified group differences.

The most appropriate method to confirm or disprove the significance of these observations is to carry out a well designed rigorous epidemiologic study of the health of the military members present at Khamisiyah during the demolition period. A request for research proposals for such an epidemiologic study has been published by the Department of Defense. If successful, research funding awards are expected to be made before the end of FY 1997.

POSTHEARING QUESTIONS FROM SENATOR JEFFORDS TO THE PRESIDENTIAL ADVISORY COMMITTEE ON GULF WAR VETERANS' ILLNESSES AND THE RESPONSES

Question 1. Your Committee determined that there is no one link between the symptoms experienced and the variety of risk factors in the Theater and urged that more research be undertaken. In your view are the planned VA projects or the current research projects underway adequate until we hear their conclusions or are there more projects that need to be undertaken?

Answer. The Advisory Committee concluded the governments current research portfolio on Gulf War veterans' illnesses—funded by VA, DOD, and HHS—is appropriately weighted toward epidemiologic studies and studies on stress-related disorders that are more likely to improve our understanding of Gulf War veterans' illnesses. We concluded that, for the most part, the governments prioritization process has worked. We recommend that any new research funds be directed toward research in: long-term health effects from stress, long-term health effects from low level exposure to chemical warfare agents, and synergistic effects of pyridostigmine bromide with other Gulf War risk factors.

Question 2. As you know, with the exception of Spina Bifida cases, the VA lacks the authority to provide benefits or services on the basis of adverse health effects in children. Based on the evidence you reviewed, how helpful would a granting of this authority be in assisting veterans and their families?

Answer. The Advisory Committee concluded that—based on biological implausibility and epidemiologic data to date—it is unlikely exposures in the Gulf War theater are responsible for birth defects of children born to veterans. Nevertheless, the Advisory Committee was concerned that if a future service connection related to reproductive matters was scientifically established for Gulf War veterans, or any other veterans, benefits and compensation still could not flow to affected parties, Therefore, we recommended that, as a general policy matter, the government conduct a thorough review of its policies concerning reproductive health and seek statutory authority to treat veterans and *their families* for service-connected problems in this regard. We emphasize, especially, that genetic counseling should be provided either via VA treatment facilities or referral—to assist veterans and their families who have reproductive concerns stemming from military service.

CORRESPONDENCE FROM SENATOR ROCKEFELLER TO DEPUTY SECRETARY OF DEFENSE JOHN D. WHITE

United States Senate

COMMITTEE ON VETERANS' AFFAIRS
WASHINGTON, DC 20510–6375

December 6, 1996

The Honorable John D. White
Deputy Secretary of Defense
The Pentagon
Washington, DC 20301-1010

Dear Deputy Secretary White:

I remain extremely concerned about the inability of the Department of Defense to recover missing pages of the military Nuclear, Biologic, Chemical (NBC) logs maintained during the Persian Gulf War, and the resulting appearance, real or illusory, that the Department is withholding information from the American public.

In light of these failures, it is imperative that you release the Executive Officer logs (XO Logs) maintained by General Norman Schwarzkopf in the Gulf between August 1990 and August 1991. The Schwarzkopf XO Logs contain very detailed notes taken by military personnel, an Executive Officer assigned to the General, for the express purpose of making a contemporaneous record of every meeting and briefing, and during every conversation and encounter in the Gulf in any way related to the War.

It is my understanding that the XO Logs were stored on three computer diskettes, with both classified and unclassified versions, and that numerous copies were maintained by not only General Schwarzkopf, but in addition others, including his Executive Officer(s), Petty Officer, CENTCOM, the Chief of Staff for Intelligence, and various Air Force personnel. Reportedly, these XO Logs were maintained for the express purpose of assisting the General in writing his memoirs after the War, and were, in fact, ultimately used for that purpose. Now, surely, these records are of critical importance, in light of the missing military NBC logs, if we are ever to shed light on what really happened in the Gulf.

I question the technical interpretation of the law that these records were personal property belonging to the General, but regardless, there is no question that the Schwarzkopf XO Logs would provide extremely valuable information about the war that has somehow disappeared from the official NBC logs.

The Honorable John D. White
December 6, 1996
Page 2

It is incumbent upon the Pentagon to release these Schwarzkopf XO LOGS into the public domain at once. I request that you provide me a complete unredacted copy of the XO Log, and in writing, a full accounting of the investigation of the Schwarzkopf XO Logs, including the following information:

1. Who has possession and control of all copies of the XO Logs at this time, both the classified and unclassified versions?

2. Has General Schwarzkopf been requested to provide copies of the XO Logs to the Defense Department for the purposes of the Persian Gulf War illness investigation?

3. The names, full identification, and present whereabouts of each and every person assigned to provide recordkeeping services to the General in the Gulf, and those who subsequently provided support services to the General during the entire time following the war that he was engaged in writing his Persian Gulf War memoirs.

4. Have each of the persons identified above been interviewed with regard to their involvement with the Schwarzkopf XO Logs? If so, please provide a full report of all that was garnished from that investigation.

Deputy Secretary White, I know you are committed to a full investigation of all facets of the Persian Gulf illnesses. In light of the missing military logs from the Gulf, it is imperative that you take all possible steps to recover and review the Schwarzkopf diaries. I look forward to your response.

Sincerely,

Jay Rockefeller

John D. Rockefeller IV
Ranking Minority Member